Brain Flowers

Brain Flowers
Ten Keys to Awakening in the Real World

Johnny Scifo

Brain Flowers: Ten Keys to Awakening in the Real World

Copyright ©2024 by Johnny Scifo

All rights reserved. This book or parts thereof may not be reproduced in any form, stored in any retrieval system, or transmitted in any form by any means—electronic, mechanical, photocopy, recording, or otherwise—without prior written permission of the publisher, except as provided by United States of America copyright law. For permission requests, write to the publisher, at CreativeScifo@gmail.com

Disclaimer: The author has made every attempt to provide information that is accurate and complete, but this book is not intended as a substitute for professional medical advice. This book is not meant to be used, nor should it be used, to diagnose or treat any medical or psychological condition. Readers are advised to consult their own medical advisors whose responsibility it is to determine the condition of, and best treatment for, the reader.

Printed in the USA

First Edition

ISBN: 979-8-9875618-0-5 (Paperback)
ISBN: 979-8-9875618-1-2 (eBook)

Library of Congress Control Number: 2024914787

Cover and interior formatting by Becky's Graphic Design®, LLC
www.BeckysGraphicDesign.com

for those who are willing to do the work,

but need a little help where to start.

CONTENTS

	Preface	ix
	Introduction	1
CHAPTER 1	Honesty	9
CHAPTER 2	Nourishment	23
CHAPTER 3	Rest	35
CHAPTER 4	Exercise	47
CHAPTER 5	Meditation	59
CHAPTER 6	Curiosity	73
CHAPTER 7	Relationships	83
CHAPTER 8	Responsibility	97
CHAPTER 9	Acceptance	111
CHAPTER 10	Generosity	121
	Thank You	135
APPENDIX I	Homegrown Retreats	139
APPENDIX II	Recommended Resources	161
	About the Author	167

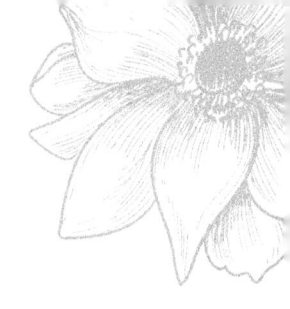

PREFACE

AS A CHILD, I was the tallest kid in class. By age thirteen, I reached six feet tall, the same height I stand today as an adult. I know that most mothers would view this as a blessing, since I was not bullied in school and was easily remembered by my teachers. But the unforeseeable side effect of being so tall at such a young age was that I rarely knew what it meant to feel small—so I fell in love with great forests, valleys, and mountains, where I could be physically insignificant in their presence. The awe that nature continues to inspire in me is unmatched by any other influence.

My teachers would often put me in the back of the class so no one would have to struggle to see around my large frame. I am blessed to be the kind of person that comprehends quickly and didn't need the repetitions characteristic of early schooling. I spent a lot of my time in the back row staring out at the trees, remaining half present at my desk and half in another realm. The shamans say that to be a healer, you must have one foot in the spiritual world and the other grounded in the material reality we all share. This allows the healer to be sensitive to subtle changes, to listen and absorb the details, continuously acting mindfully to bring the future into being. The furthest back I can recall having such a sensitivity within myself is instinctively feeling the precise moment when the teacher was switching subjects and I knew it was time to pay attention again, though my thoughts still flew above the trees with the birds squawking outside.

Crows were the ubiquitous birds of my childhood; their caws and yips woke me up regularly. In hindsight, they were my first spiritual friends, leading me to realize how much more there is to life than the mundane pursuit of material things. Even now, every time I see crows, they seem to have the mystical ability to make time stop. In our busy world, such an impact is truly magical. I take their presence as a sign they are checking on me to ensure I am still on my path, still doing my practice, bringing me back to the present moment.

It was such an instance on a personal retreat into the mountains, when a group of crows soared past me, that I decided to finish this book once and for all. Despite feeling at the top of my game at work, solid in my new marriage, and mentally preparing to become a father, I was far away from the person I thought I was going to be when I grew up. As a breeze hugged and slipped around me, I realized how much I was still a child and how we all need things that keep bringing us back to our roots.

For nearly two decades, I have been a spiritual seeker. I became a certified yoga teacher and trained to the highest distinction a teacher can acquire. I now train other teachers in my unique blend of music and meditation practices, since I am also a sound healer and herbalist, and I have gone through shamanic initiation. I did this training all while inheriting a family business and maintaining it for the fourth generation. My meditation practice started as a way to deal with my bouts of anxiety and depression. I am the walking, talking proof that even if you are a little nuts, you can find peace in the chaos of this world. But I think the most notable part of my journey is that I never had the opportunity to completely disappear from modern life and come back "enlightened." Throughout my years of practice and training, I have either been studying or working full time.

My yoga practice began in college, when I was studying abroad in Australia. One day, I saw a bunch of gray-haired ladies doing yoga on the beach. Laughing, smiling, and shockingly flexible, these women exuded vitality. I found them wonderfully inspiring, as I sat there chubby, hungover, and chronically fatigued. I needed something to shake me up, give me some mojo. I decided right then I would commit to a basic yoga routine when I got back to the States. I was not much for cardio or lifting weights, and I liked the idea of doing something with the potential for such longevity.

That single moment ignited a hidden passion that led to seven years of practicing in secret, what I like to think of as my first phase of spiritual revolution. At that point, I didn't know that yoga studios existed (they were not nearly as popular back then), and even if I did, it's unlikely I would have had the courage to work out in public anyway. I hid my mat under my bed and practiced in my dorm room while my roommate was at class. I began to seriously think about what I was eating and how partying disrupted my sleep schedule. This minimal yet honest awareness grounded me enough to get my economics degree and get into law school with a scholarship. A year later, I would drop out and go to design school instead. This led to major family disappointments and repercussions, as I pursued being a professional photographer and graphic designer by day and a musician by night. I had been playing the drums onstage since age ten and thought I was "living my truth" working as a freelancer instead of being a law student. But while I was (barely) paying the bills, I *was* beating myself up in an unsustainable way. My father noticed and invited me to come and work with him while I figured things out, or in his words, *get your act together and grow up once and for all.* It was tough, mostly because I was doing well enough in the music scene to feel like I had momentum, but I conceded that working a 9-to-5 job would be better for my finances.

It didn't take long for my double life to really bum me out. I kept my ambitions alive by setting up a summer tour under "make or break" terms. I would go to work during the week so as not to shirk my responsibilities, fly out after work on Friday, rock a Saturday performance, and fly back on Sunday. *I'll sleep on the plane or sleep at my desk. Just make it work! Sacrifice! This is the dream!* It was a temporary setup, and I was getting at least some of the best of both worlds, making money and music. I decided to try and grind it out.

With sixteen weeks of shows set up, I made it to week seven before I crashed and burned. Sick, exhausted, and much too casual about what substances were entering my body, it took multiple hospital visits before I got the message: *there are certain things that are not meant to be*, no matter how much energy you throw at them or how much you are willing to sacrifice.

I will forever remember my rock-bottom moment. It's not necessary for all of us to have a "dark night of the soul" in order to find our way. But since I am a stubborn SOB, I needed the universe to beat me to the point of ego-death before I hung it up. The funny thing about such moments of total failure and rejection is that when you let go of who you thought you were meant to be, it reopens a world of possibilities. Feeling depleted, I acknowledged that my yoga practice was still my bedrock, and that was where I would begin again.

The second phase of my spiritual revolution began with yoga teacher training a decade ago, seven years after I first got on a mat. When I graduated, my mentors implored me to teach. I had really only gone into training to become more knowledgeable about my practice. I was still working for my dad, and even throughout training, I really didn't think that I'd ever teach. My practice was very personal and private for me—I had yet to attend a yoga class outside of mandatory classwork. But some of my outward progress was now becoming obvious, and people were asking me what I was up to these days. To be fair, I *had* lost seventy pounds, a quarter of my body weight at the time. My whole food, plant-based eating habits had cleared up my skin too. I was also walking on a cloud, because at the studio where I was training I had just met the woman I would later call my wife. I was using my twenty-plus years of musical experience to tap into meditative states with an ease I did not fully comprehend. Whatever I was digging into was powerful, and more than once I was told by my mentors to pursue it fervently, while proceeding cautiously.

I started to write as a personal survival tool. I noticed some behavioral patterns, then jotted advice to my future self, in case I was in the same spot again (which often happened). The ideas typically started as wild tirades, but with additional life experience, practice, and wisdom, I distilled my journal into learned lessons. I kept reading anything I could about wellness, meditation, and the space where neuroscience discoveries mix with ancient wisdom.

I recorded some meditation music in my home studio, and after sharing it in local yoga circles, it was picked up by a small app called Insight Timer. At the time, they were just starting out and couldn't pay me, but they hoped that these early efforts would pay dividends down the line. Since I had failed to meet my musical aspirations before and had no teaching aspirations to fulfill, it was no big deal to me to give away my music for free. My philosophy was *Share it! Spread peace! For the children!*

It got around, and fast. My skill set from being such a pleasure-seeking monster as a younger man, tempered by my new wisdom through training and studying, created something that was relaxing and useful to others. I began leading small classes using my unique blend of music and meditation techniques, which quickly added up to thousands of students at yoga festivals, leading retreats, and sharing my take on meditation, music, and neuroscience with educators in both academia and spiritual circles, including Lululemon, Kripalu, the Rubin Museum, Ramapo College, and SUNY New Paltz.

And that was just on the weekends. During the week, I was gradually taking the reins of our family business from my father. My awareness in my yoga practice positively translated into my performance at work too. My retreat weekends were restorative for me as well, and I was not burning out this time around. I continued to write as a practice to keep myself engaged, taking notes on core similarities as I trained in other healing modalities. Bouncing from Yoga to Soto Zen to the Peruvian Shamans, with many a stopover in between, I scoured through hundreds of books, lectures, and resources, and I noticed how widely different cultures shared similar ethics for living in harmony with ourselves and our surroundings and that many of these overlapping teachings were backed by science.

Then the pandemic came, and I pretty much lost everything I had going as a yoga teacher. The studio where I was primarily teaching went bankrupt, and other studios in the area had closed indefinitely. Festivals and retreats halted and the great majority never returned. The magazines for whom I wrote articles also closed up shop. I tried teaching online, but being a guy that utilizes the energy of a room onstage and spends most of his spare time in the woods, talking through a screen indoors next to the Wi-Fi... well, that was a tough transition for me. But I didn't want my work to end there, because it felt unfinished. So I began retracing through notes and my workshops, and the main tenets that have shaped my journey and successes became very clear. I called them the ten keys.

The following teachings are for *you* and not about me or my experience. My journey is mine, yours is yours. The only reason I share my story at all is to let you know that I am not preaching from on high. It's not theoretical for me. I did the work. It was hard to transition, but now that I have, I am happy. I am *not* trying to convince you to be like me. I want you to thrive as the best version of *you*. I can help plant the seeds through these teachings, but you have to water the soil and grow the flowers. Most of these teachings relate back to our brains, and science has shown us that our brains are malleable through our experiences. This means that the choices we make literally change our brains, for better or worse. We choose how our minds grow, how the brain flowers.

PREFACE

I can remember when I first began taking care of myself properly, I did not have a lot of energy to put into reading long books about awakening, riddles of old monks and nuns, or varying translations of Sanskrit mantras. This is the book that I needed back then, that gets right to the point of offering some solutions, yet leaves enough room for the reader to come to their own conclusions. Honestly, the people who often need the lessons the most are the ones least likely to sit down and do the work. So, I wrote a book of lessons that can apply to anyone, anywhere, and made it short and dense on purpose. I wrote it in the Western tongues of science and secularity to keep it accessible to the widest audience, with a few exceptions for words that defy translation. My hope is that it can be read and reread, with different lessons revealing themselves when the time is right.

This is not an attempt to form a new religion, nor am I anyone's guru. This is a book about what it means to be human and how to survive well. For me, this is the starting point to an awakened life—to live fully realized, and enjoy it.

Thank you for sharing in my journey.

I wish you all the luck in yours.

Meditation Practice in 100 Words

Set a timer in a quiet place.
Straight spine, sitting on a cushion or chair.
Support body weight, do not lean.
Relax. Get comfortable.

Breathe deeply, in and out through the nose (ideally).
Eyes closed or staring downward without focusing.
Hear the room, don't disappear.

Focus on the breath.
Inhale. Exhale.
In. Out.

Breathe deeper. Notice the breath.
Steady? Shaky? Tight? Relaxed?
No judgments. Just notice.
Inhale. Exhale.
In. Out.

When the mind wanders off, notice where it goes,
but do not linger there.
Come back to the breath.
Inhale. Exhale.
In. Out.

Sit until timer finishes.
Bow in gratitude.
Repeat.

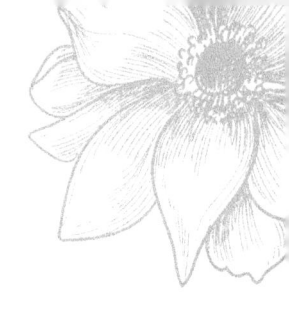

INTRODUCTION

LET US BEGIN BY considering meditation as a state of being, rather than exclusively as a practice. Usually we think of meditation as a seated cross-legged monk in lotus posture, perhaps humming or chanting. This describes the formal practice of meditation, when we sit quietly, follow our breath or a sound, and try to enter a peaceful state of mind. It is the mental state that we are practicing, not the sitting. The cushion, the quiet, and the posture are all meant to ease us more readily into the meditation mind space. It is not a blissed-out or zombie state. Meditation can be more accurately described as fully aware, in the present moment, and perceiving reality without judgments.

There are many meditation practice techniques, as different cultures have found their own doorways into this peaceful, connected state of being. The good news is they all lead to the same place. Exploring different techniques and finding the right fit is part of the journey.

The best technique is the one that you are willing to continue practicing.

But meditation is not reserved for sitting practice alone. The peaceful state of being we cultivate on the cushion must continue to be expressed through our actions. We are in meditation while cutting vegetables, waiting at a traffic light, even when taking criticism from a loved one. The process of learning to express meditation in our actions is called *awakening.* The awakening process is gradual, as we continue to mindfully bring our attention to our words and behaviors and choose right actions over harmful and ignorant alternatives. There are lightning rod insights, but these moments are not magical. They are a product of doing the necessary spiritual work. As we continue to bring conscious attention to our actions, the awakening process opens us up to greater possibilities for love, peace, and abundance.

The full expression of awakening—where we successfully operate in meditation through all our actions—is called *enlightenment.* The debate continues whether it is our natural state to which we must return or an attainment of spiritual wisdom. Yet even if we view enlightenment as only an ideal, it is a great aspiration. Our awakening path will be a process of choosing the right actions, regardless of the conditions.

Everyone has their own journey toward awakening, but for many of us it begins by acknowledging some imbalance in our lives, one that is likely making us suffer. Suffering is caused when you experience pain and then resist it. Pain is a natural form of communication, one that makes us stop because harm is befalling us. Pain by itself is not a bad thing; it is often a warning. But it's the way we react to pain that does us in. When we dwell on this pain or ignore it, we suffer. Think of it this way: It would be silly to continue to complain about a stubbed toe days after it has healed or to ignore a bleeding wound in hopes it just gets better without bandaging it. But often, this is precisely what we do with our emotions. The unfortunate reality is that our nervous systems do not distinguish between emotional and physical pain. By operating from a state of meditation, we can see pain clearly without getting attached to it or resisting it. When we better understand our circumstances and environment, we allow ourselves to gather all the facts before reacting. By slowing down and operating with a deeper connection, we reduce the risk of causing conflict and proceed with correct actions. We are most likely to maintain our meditation when we feel balanced and synchronized in mind, body, and spirit.

Within our physical bodies, internal systems maintain homeostasis, a balanced state that keeps us running optimally; and the best point or range is called equilibrium. A simple example of homeostasis is internal temperature regulation. When we run a fever, our temperature spikes out of equilibrium range, and we begin to sweat and cool down. We don't have to think, "sweat, cool down," because internal autonomic systems, outside of our conscious control, are working the gearshifts.

Our conscious awareness—what we *do* control—is only a part of the overall human experience. This is a good thing, otherwise we'd have to consciously remember to breathe! Yet your conscious actions will have a direct impact on your energy levels. Acting with awareness leads to decisions that simultaneously support our state of meditation and homeostasis.

As our world becomes increasingly stimulating, particularly through technology, many of us need to take additional actions to stay in balance. We may need specific practices to ensure we continue to stay in meditation. The process of awakening is a wonderful template for addressing the pressures of modernity and maintaining a healthy well-being, but that is only the start of a spiritual journey. When we feel better, we do better.

The revolution is from within. The answer is not *out there* somewhere but exactly where we are, here and now. Like most of you, I live outside of monastic life in the "real world." I am not immune to the challenges, nor do I hold some romanticized view of the past. Even though our world is interconnected through technology, it's also been turned upside down because of it. A lot of our outer circumstances have changed, but biologically, we are mostly the same as our ancestors.

The following ten keys to awakening are not intellectual but practical, down to earth, and focused on the human experience we all share. After years of reading everything from scripture to self-help books, I feel these are the subjects of what it means to be human. They do not require any alterations to belief systems because they do not require any beliefs. Unlike other spiritual works that try to persuade the reader toward a particular view, this is a template for thinking about spiritual practice in everyday living, leaving space for the reader to tailor their individual practices.

At the end of each chapter, I'll offer a series of questions to jump-start an inner dialogue about where you are in the present moment. You'll also find a reference section, with a guide to creating your own spiritual retreats at home and where I list my favorite resources, specific to each key, for deeper investigation when the appropriate time arises. Don't rush. Wisdom is timeless. It is not wisdom that changes, but rather it's *we* who do the changing. I have humbly attempted to organize these teachings, both spiritual and scientific, to serve our collective awakening.

The meditation master Chögyam Trungpa Rinpoche said the great spiritual teachers of the future will come from America because they will be the first to have faced the latest human challenges regarding technology and materialism. As one of those teachers, I take up this mantle to share what I have learned, cast light on the problems we share, and offer the solutions that have served me greatly in my awakening journey. I love how a lit candle can continue to emblaze a thousand additional candles without the expense of its own flame. In the same way, I pray this work brings you light.

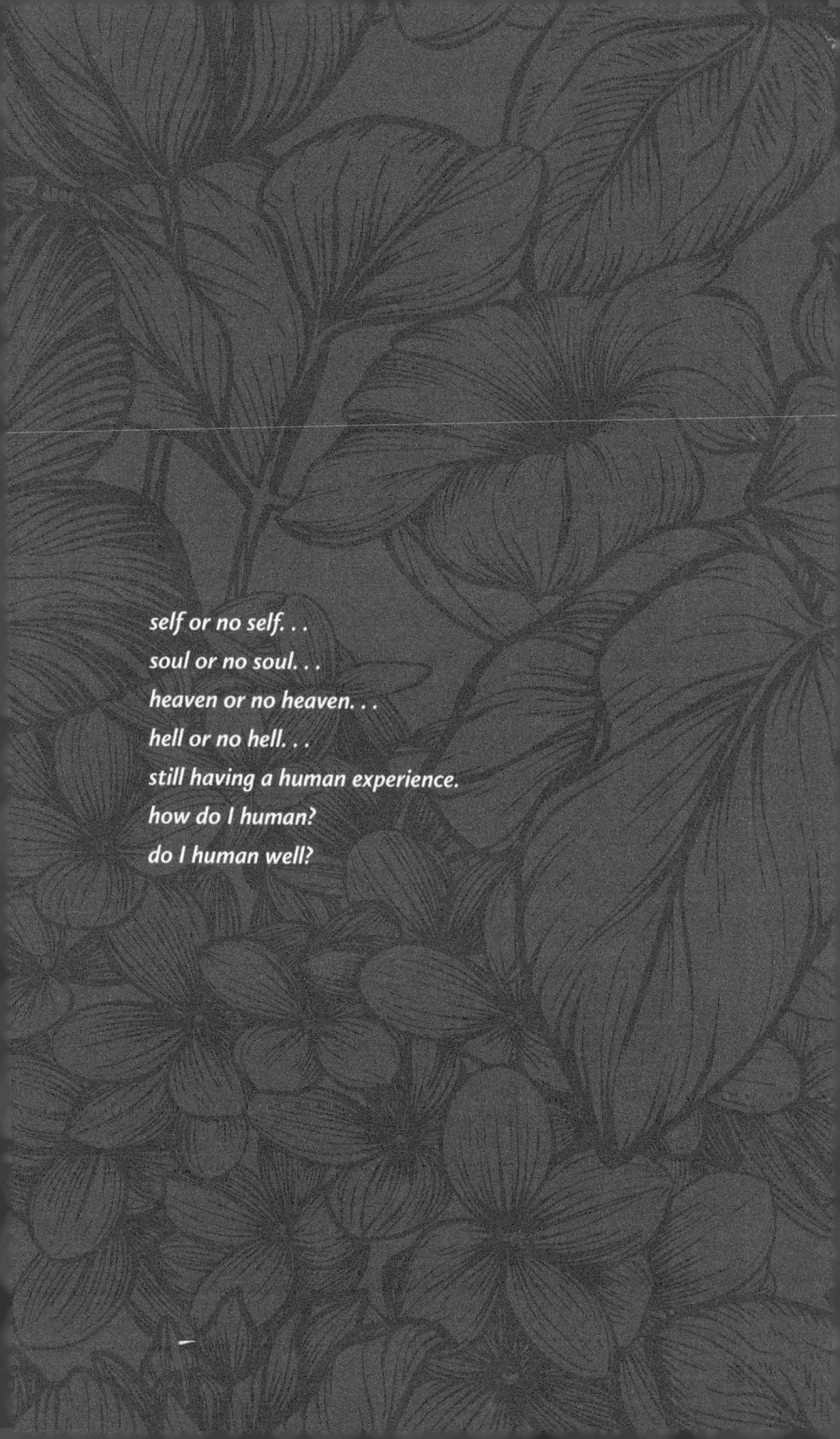

self or no self...
soul or no soul...
heaven or no heaven...
hell or no hell...
still having a human experience.
how do I human?
do I human well?

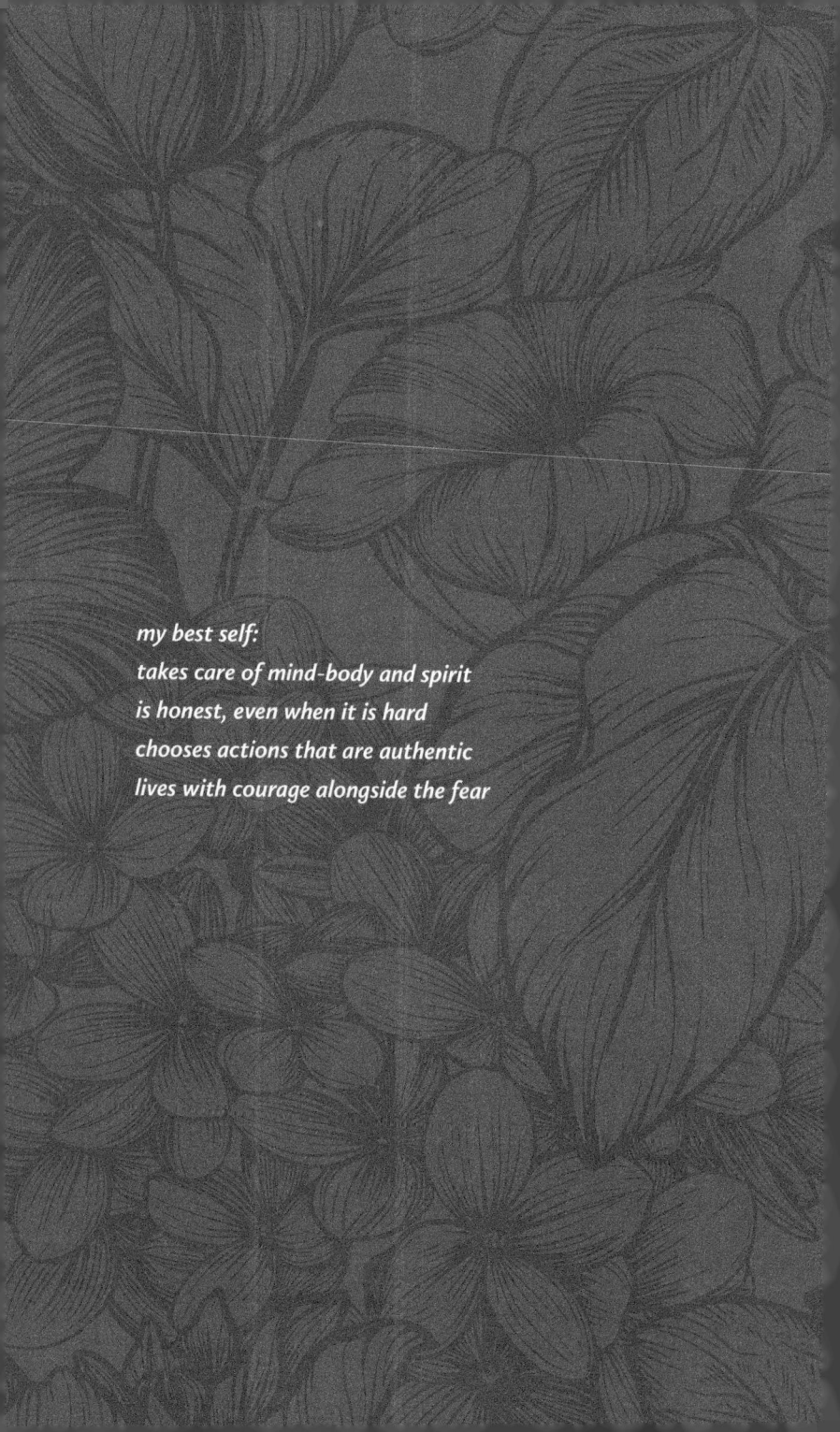

my best self:
takes care of mind-body and spirit
is honest, even when it is hard
chooses actions that are authentic
lives with courage alongside the fear

1

HONESTY

***SPIRITUAL MATERIALISM* MANIFESTS IN** a variety of forms. It is the attempt to compartmentalize spirituality into neat little boxes and keep it separate from everyday living. It is revering any spiritual culture so much that it becomes viewed as unattainable or something we cannot participate in ourselves. It is wanting something good in return for being a spiritual person, a sort of entitlement gained for keeping up the practice. But spirituality cannot be kept in a box or on a pedestal, to be pulled out only when necessary or when tradition calls. It has to become part of our ordinary experience, in every present moment. It is not enough to simply understand spiritual teachings logically or agree with the principles in theory; they must become embodied in our actions. Awakening is the process of learning to operate in meditation in all of our actions, to walk through life with grace and ease, regardless of the conditions. This will continue to seem impossible if we limit our meditation to a practice of sitting with our eyes closed, rather than seeing it as a peaceful state of being, always available to us.

The first step requires us to eliminate any barriers between our spiritual practice and daily lives—including the parts of life that are unglamourous, mundane, and repetitive. In our filtered world on screens, these parts of our lives are continuously underrepresented or flat out ignored. Consequently, we chase happiness and hyper-stimulating experiences, instead of cultivating contentment. We seek to fulfill our desires, putting all our efforts into some version of the future, instead of being present. We want good vibes only, all the time, as if getting rid of all the undesirable parts of our lives will lock us in a perpetual state of delight.

While it is natural to seek pleasure and avoid pain, no one can live a painless reality all the time. Often we hide from our pain instead of facing it with dignity. Many of us waste too much effort swimming against the current, instead of going with the flow. Many of us carry too many anchors while trying to stay afloat. Whether it is our material possessions or emotional baggage, each of us has our *stuff*. A lot of *stuff* drags our energy levels down as we move through the day, whether or not we are conscious about the way we carry it.

Our brains are supercomputers, trying to forecast the future by drawing from our past experiences. Yet by coming to stillness through our meditation practice, you can begin to witness the ping-ponging back and forth between memories and predictions. We cannot shut our brains off. We must become friends with our minds and their processes. Simply put, we are *not* our thoughts. Thoughts are the result of our brains trying to interpret our surroundings and make accurate predictions based on the sensory cues we are receiving. Creating thoughts is simply what the brain does. You may hear about how thoughts become things, but can you imagine if your darkest, oddest, or creepiest thoughts became manifestations? Thoughts only become things if we put energy into them. Being honest about where we put our energy is an important part of the awakening process.

Meditation sitting practice is an opportunity to witness where our energy gravitates. On the cushion, we notice our thoughts and we let them go, continuously returning to the breath or object of focus, simply being present. But at some point, we must acknowledge what we are noticing on the cushion and make the appropriate modifications. Perhaps we notice we are boiling with impatience, or we keep replaying a mistake over and over in our minds. These are the inner thoughts that use our energy, with or without our consent. To make friends with our minds is to notice these thoughts honestly and not to overreact or get defensive when they are not flattering.

When you view your situation with honesty, then you can make a plan. The plan may be as simple as doing nothing and letting things continue to take their natural course, but you sit in the situation differently. You shift from being a spectator unaware of what is to come to an actor working quietly. To the outside world, you may seem the same, perhaps a bit more relaxed. But inside you have a clear view into your inner dialogue, can evaluate your thoughts objectively, and cut them off mercilessly when necessary. Sometimes noticing a bad habit is enough to clear things up. But sometimes, it is just the beginning of a long, dragged-out fight with inner demons. Either way, each day offers us a blank slate. Do we begin by chiseling the woes of yesterday or open ourselves to the fresh inspiration available today? It takes conscious awareness to move through life in this way, with eyes figuratively (and sometimes literally) wide open, which is why we equate it to being awake, as opposed to being asleep, on autopilot, or unconscious.

You have everything you need right here and now to awaken. It may not feel this way, especially when desires are still taking the wheel. Often, we confuse our desires with our needs because our emotions are so strong. We feel like, *all I need is this thing, or person, or situation, to work out and then I will be happy / fine / complete.* That is where our focus goes, often damaging something else in the process. Too many of us make harmful and unnecessary sacrifices along the way to fulfill such desires. But the revolution is from within, and it is determined by our inner state, not conditions or resources outside of ourselves. Many of us have had the experience of getting exactly what we wanted, only to find out it was not as fulfilling as we initially believed. To dial in on what is truly important, try this exercise:

Let us say in an hour, I am going to pick you up and we are not going to be back for a month. Your bags are already packed for you. All you need to do is handle your personal affairs. What are the responsibilities that immediately come to mind that you would have to make arrangements for? What would you leave hanging in the balance or drop without a second thought? What stresses you out just thinking about it? In our interdependent society, this exercise illustrates where we are connected. The real question is, which of these things are really important and which stressors are self-imposed?

Reflecting on our habits reveals the areas of our lives where we are thriving, as well as where we would be wiser to preserve our energy or change our approach. Chances are, there are things you are doing well, things that make life easier, bring joy, and contribute to your well-being. But we may be less skillful in handling other aspects of our lives, and consequently, they are using more energy than they deserve, causing imbalances. Many of us jam our lives with activities and our *stuff* until it feels like we are going to burst, keeping ourselves in constant states of distracted busyness. But a full schedule does not necessarily equate to a good life.

A good life is defined by your ability to live authentically. Authenticity comes from being comfortable with who we are and operating with confidence that allows us to be honest about our feelings and circumstances. It requires a certain amount of spaciousness, but it does not include any guarantee of attaining our goals or creating the dream life. Living authentically is deeper than that—realizing that there is nothing to attain and just appreciating the mystery of the here and now. Often, we are too focused on creating our lives, instead of simply living them.

When we try too hard to generate a situation or outcome, we get caught up in expectations. Expectations are not based in honesty; they are based in desire. It is natural to have preferences, but when we become attached to a particular outcome, problems usually follow. Our attachments often blind us to the truth. We must be honest when there is only a tiny possibility of a situation working out the way we want, no matter how passionately our desire may burn. Teenage romantic crushes are often fertile grounds for this lesson. Many eager hearts have been broken only to realize later that all the signs of doom were there. But at the time, something kept us from seeing the situation clearly. Perhaps we did not take in all the details, or denied the whole picture, or omitted facts contrary to the desired outcome. Whatever the case, our version was incorrect, our expectations were unfulfilled, and we were "crushed."

You must ask yourself if you are wearing any rose-colored glasses—judgments, desires, *stuff*—that may be keeping you from seeing the situation clearly. Because while after a certain age you can laugh about those rosy glasses that led to teenaged unrequited love, we are likely still clinging to juvenile fantasies in other areas of our lives. We may be wiser to admit if something is not meant to be, rather than sacrificing ourselves by committing to such a narrow path for success. Positive thinking is wonderful when it is appropriate. But when it is not, optimism can be a form of denial. Too many of us believe that wishing for something and staying positive that it will work out is enough. It is not. Instead, we must see things as they are, without our judgments or desires attached to them. With that clarity, we need to apply the appropriate effort too. This is practicing honesty.

When we begin to sift through our *stuff*, we often become aware of how carelessly we have previously existed. We may find ourselves doing certain things for logical or practical reasons but now we notice they are not good emotional fits for us; or just the opposite, we have prioritized good emotional fits that still lead to other problems. There may be an ugly quality to being so honest, but if we continue to live in denial, we will refrain from opening up and living with more ease. We all make poor choices. Sometimes it is no big deal, and we can resolve our issues by mindfully bringing our attention back to the present moment and cleaning up our acts. But there are other patterns that may need more tough love to correct—including admitting there is a problem in the first place.

Until we unpack our *stuff*, the way forward may feel imbalanced, especially when it is not obvious where the discomfort is coming from or what to do about it. If you dump your whole emotional bag on the floor (and some of us may have to), you'd better be prepared to deal with the mess all at once. Modern life does not usually give you adequate space for this kind of dumping. For most of us, we will be more effective by prioritizing what in our lives gives us stability and continue to build upon those areas. The journey is one step at a time.

Begin by unpacking one item at a time. Bring each item to a place of rest (even if only temporarily) before moving on to the next one. For the parts of our life that we can identify as problematic, we must be resolute in taking action, or else nothing will change. By seeing things as they are, instead of how we wish them to be, we may recognize that there is a limit to what we can control in a given situation. This honesty can illuminate what our efforts can accomplish and where we may be spinning our wheels. Only we know where our daily efforts and attention are spent.

Being honest with yourself is primarily about the relationship between how you are feeling and what you are doing. It isn't a check-in about how we are doing compared to anyone else or how well we are achieving our desires. Comparisons are useless because *your* growth is based exclusively on *your* efforts and actions. There is no universal guide for how to live, but we recognize that we live within the context of our values, shared in part through religion, community, country, and more. The trickier questions can only be answered by us individually.

When we begin to notice ourselves with new awareness, we can become very critical of this mental activity in which no one else participates. No matter what level of effort we put forward to show the world, it will be useless if we are lying to ourselves. Life is not perfect. Most people are so wrapped up in their own *stuff* they are not paying attention to us anyway. We are only lying to ourselves in these moments.

Build upon the good in life right now, in your immediate world, in the ways that *you* can control. Acting with more awareness instantly improves situations, followed by skillful actions. If we put in honest effort and attention, we can make space for the things in our lives that we wish to manifest. Less is more. By reducing our personal distractions and self-imposed stressors, we reduce the likelihood of causing accidental harm and focus on what is really important to us and what authentically supports the life we are consciously experiencing.

REFLECTIONS

What comprises my *stuff*? What am I doing about it?

Am I being honest with myself about my efforts?

Is there anything I am intentionally ignoring that I should address?

What are the supportive areas in my life that I can build upon?

What areas of my life feel smooth and calm?

Is there anything that I am dreading, holding on to, or obsessing over unnecessarily?

Am I being patient or waiting around for something that is unlikely to happen?

Do I truly feel overwhelmed or am I continuing to procrastinate?

Where am I mentally—here or somewhere else? And how about emotionally?

What am I craving, and is this craving also nourishing?

What areas of my life have little or no flexibility?

i am all elements,
balanced
silent
and always present.

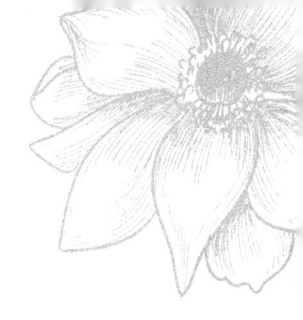

2

NOURISHMENT

THROUGH OUR FOOD WE maintain our health and stamina, yet the anatomical processes that convert our calories into energy are handled by systems outside of our conscious attention. Once the food goes down, we are no longer in control of it. But we are always in control of what we put into our mouths.

Eating is a good place to begin viewing ourselves with honesty, because it is an activity that we repeat daily. It is a conscious act. We cannot subconsciously eat, even if we munch mindlessly. Every meal can be an opportunity to pause, reflect, and if necessary, hit the reset button. Our healthiest food choices for our bodies are largely influenced by our heritage and genetics, making it nearly impossible to prescribe the ultimate diet to guarantee well-being. Consequently, it is a risky subject to be definitive about because it is so subjective. Food also has a lot of our *stuff* attached to it—from positive memories of relatives and their special recipes to negative habits of numbing out during emotional binge eating. Food can enhance your mood when you are sluggish or cranky, but it can also lead to imbalances like sugar crashes and indigestion. Whether eating for pleasure or fuel, each choice can compound positively or negatively upon the last.

Eating well means consuming nutrients that react positively with our bodies. Finding your personal recipes for success is a lifelong practice. Our bodies change as we age, and the recipe book is constantly being edited. The ingredients most likely to withstand the test of time are local, seasonal, and organic. Beyond that, I think we can all agree that we do not want to poison ourselves.

Lectins are plant poisons: a plant's natural chemical protection to keep away bugs and predators. We have resistance to most lectins that we consume but we can become ill by consuming too many at once, especially in foods in which we are not locally exposed or well adapted. A lot of the plants we eat have lectins until the plant fully ripens its seeds and flowers or grows to a certain maturity. Lectins recede when the plant wishes animals to interact with it. An easy example is a green apple turning red once ripe. When we wait to witness the signals from nature and pick our foods only when they are ripe, the lectins will have receded out of the edible parts, and they become a nonissue.

But in the modern world, produce is often picked prematurely so it can appear ripe by the time it reaches the faraway destination where it will be sold. This is especially likely for fresh produce in the off-season (which is why we often see organic produce from other countries in the winter). The problem is, lectins are only naturally removed by the plant itself, not through time alone. If picked too early, the lectins are trapped in the premature fruit. The apple does not actually ripen to maturity, it simply turns red, often through synthetic processes. Then when you pick it up at the grocery, it says organic from another country, it is nice and red, but it is still filled with lectins! Processed foods are also problematic, as companies ship ingredients from around the world to maintain consistent flavor profiles all year. Here and there, lectins are no big deal. But consume enough, and it becomes a pattern of inflammation, fatigue, gas, and nausea. Increased exposure can even lead to more harmful conditions, including leaky gut.

You can avoid lectin issues completely by eating seasonal, fresh, whole foods and sourcing them locally. Local farmers naturally pick foods at the proper seasonal maturity schedule because the food does not have far to travel, greatly reducing the likelihood of lectins by honoring the cues from nature in real time, not arrival time. Get to know your food supply chain, hopefully including the farmers, and learn what is in season each month. Like my longtime friend Guy Jones of Blooming Hill Organic Farm says, "Don't buy food from strangers!"

Food is fuel. If there are no nutrients in the fuel, it doesn't matter that you're full, your body is still seeking nutrients—which is why you can feel stuffed and then be hungry thirty minutes later. The nutrient density of our food makes a difference in how much we need to eat in order to be satisfied. Our bodies use two systems to alert us when we have had enough: through physical fullness or when we have consumed enough nutrients. Slowing down when we eat can be a huge help to allow the healthier nutrient-based alert system, often referred to as satiety, to respond, especially when eating nutrient-dense food. There is a maxim to leave the table when eighty percent full in order to let satiety catch up.

Organics have more vitamins, micronutrients, and macronutrients per capita than modified or conventionally grown produce because these farmers focus on cultivating the source of the nutrients—the soil. This allows us to eat less and reduce the likelihood of digestive issues from overeating. If you don't believe me, I really encourage you to experiment and taste the difference for confirmation. With unprocessed, organic whole foods, increased flavor equals increased nutrients.

You can improve your health by noticing how you feel after each meal. Are you invigorated or ready for a nap? Quality food will make us feel energized because it is giving us nutrients to convert into energy. Poor food choices and overeating make us tired because they are throwing off the body's balancing systems, requiring more energy to digest the food than it is likely worth. Try forgoing sugar whenever possible, cutting back on gluten (not necessarily giving it up, but just cutting back on refined wheat and carbohydrate-heavy foods), and eating more whole grains and alkaline foods, particularly more leafy greens. If you have stomach issues or feel like you have indigestion regularly, alkaline foods like brussels sprouts, kale, and carrots are usually a really big help. It may take some research to find foods that qualify as local, seasonal, organic, *and* on the list of things you are willing to eat. Until then, remember the simple adage from author Michael Pollan: "Eat [real, whole] food. Mostly plants. Not too much."

Through the soil, we are all connected. In our times of technology and climate change (and most recently a global pandemic), the planet's interconnectedness is exemplified so glaringly that few of us would deny it. Many of us do not resist these connections in theory but struggle more in practice, in our behaviors.

We must awaken a stronger understanding of what our actions mean to each other, and that includes the plants and the animals around us. Let us do an exercise to illustrate this more pointedly.

As you sit down to your next meal, focus in on the ingredients. Pick one, a fruit or vegetable (for this example I will choose an apple). First, take a bite. Come to the present moment by taking in the sweet, tart flavor and fleshy, crunchy texture. Find some enjoyment in the full sensory experience: the deep red color, the crisp smell, the sounds of munching. Now let's take a moment to focus on how unique this moment is and how many beings it took to make this moment possible.

Where did the apple come from? It likely came from a market, where you picked it up and purchased it. How many people walked by that apple as it waited there for you? Even before that, someone had to put that apple on the shelf in the place that you would see it and say, *now that looks delicious.* Even before that, someone else had to pick up the apples at the farm to deliver them to the market, so they could be on display in time for you to walk by and buy them. Prior to that, someone picked that apple off a tree at the precise moment that it would be ripe enough for you to eat. That fruit only came to be after the seasonal changes of spring dew, through summer rains, and the cooling temperatures of autumn. It took years for that tree to be strong enough to even bear fruit, and it was cared for by various farmers' hands in order to be productive this year. That land may have been in the family for generations, and there have been countless apples in their orchards that have fed the families in the neighborhood. Without the community's support generations ago, none of this land would have been able to be cultivated so it could feed us today.

Countless cycles of nesting, farming, watering, fertilizing, raining, cultivating, picking, delivering, and displaying had to successfully happen for that fruit stand to be there today—through the droughts, bankruptcies, cultural wars, you name it. With this in mind, it isn't so crazy to say that it may have taken one hundred years for you to get this exact apple, from the moment the farm was founded and the first seeds planted to this moment at your table, with countless people and transactions to be completed in order for you to take this single bite, here and now. And we can go on and on, deeper into history, spreading wider to include more interconnected stories, migrations, circumstances, and lives that made this moment possible. Just start thinking about the other ingredients on your plate. Perhaps it took a million beings to make your salad?

This practice illustrates how we are all connected. We only have one planet. We cannot fathom how each of our actions are adding up altogether, so we must do our best to be mindful of each other and not cause harm. By eating locally, seasonally, and organically, we reduce our carbon footprint and the number of resources it takes to keep us healthy, while honoring the systems that directly support us.

Whatever you choose to munch, eat for your health, and not just some ideal. Choosing something like vegetarianism or veganism for spiritual purposes may seem noble, but only if it is a good fit for your body. Notice how your food choices impact the way you feel afterwards, eat more slowly, and focus inward. This is the practice of awakening: to make conscious decisions and choose the right action. Right action is not always desirous or pleasurable, and it may take a while before we get confirmation that our actions were appropriate. But we know inside when we make the right choice, even if we can only admit it to ourselves.

Let each meal serve as a source of strength. We do not need to get all our strength from a single meal. We just don't want to be hungry until the next opportunity to eat. Similarly, we can approach our awakening process in this way: bite-sized.

When we choose health over convenience, it may change the way our day is structured. It sounds simple enough, but it may not prove so easy to think about everything you put in your body, especially if you usually eat on the run. It may feel like an even bigger ask to stop all other activities to focus exclusively on nourishing ourselves during meals. But what are we more focused on, that we deem more important, than nourishing ourselves? Eat meals without distractions. Cook your own food, and connect with where it comes from. Calories are actual energy, and their source matters. Consumption is part of the human experience and we should not feel guilty about that, so long as we are mindful and not wasteful. Let the daily rituals surrounding eating become practices for awakening.

REFLECTIONS

What have I eaten over the last two days? Does anything stick out as particularly satisfying or disruptive?

How did my last meal make me feel, tired or energized?

What is the ratio of meals I eat for nutrients and foods I eat for pleasure?

Is there balance in the things that I eat?

Do I often feel bloated after eating?

How acidic is my diet?

How colorful is my plate?

What is my relationship with sugar?

How much do I waste?

NOURISHMENT

How many farmers do I know?

Do I know where my food comes from?

*growth is not always upwards.
There are times where we must lean out,
swing wide, double back,
or return attention to our roots.
It is all in the name of better reaching the light,
even if it isn't always in the direction of the sun.*

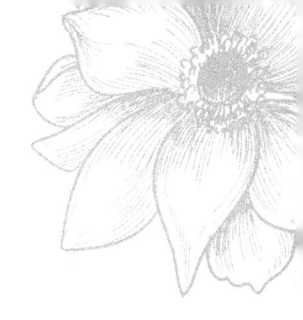

3

REST

YOU MAY BE HUMORED, or maybe even annoyed, by the nagging sense that the awakening path so far is as simple as being honest, eating well, and now, prioritizing getting a good night of sleep. But it cannot be overstated that our health is imperative to keeping up our strength to meet life's challenges openly and fearlessly. Most of us undervalue sleep. We learn very little about sleep in school, nor are we ever taught exactly how to rest. By bringing our awareness to our beds, we can ensure we fully utilize our sleep, one of our most underrated superpowers.

Throughout the day, our brains are live recording, breaking down our sensory experiences into information sent through millions of pathways called synapses, which allow information to run to various destinations and create memories. Things that we continue to bring into our awareness create stronger pathways in the brain, as we reload the memories, or repeat the experience.

Each time we repeat an action that triggers the same synapse, we make it easier to recall the information again. Perhaps you have heard that in order to master something you need to do it 10,000 times? That is an old way of saying practice makes a pathway strong and automatic. Like a river, slowly eroding the land, each time we let those thoughts run their course, we make the river a little deeper for that same thought, making it flow easier. The river takes the path of least resistance. In disaster situations we often hear emergency personnel say things like, "I didn't even think, my training just kicked in," because these pathways have been dredged deeply through training hours, which prepared them for the moment of trial.

For most of us, the pathways are less extreme. We wake up and do our morning routine while half asleep. We commute on autopilot because we take the same route every day. Have you ever checked your email and then checked it again five minutes later because you couldn't recall what you saw in your inbox? The river is dredged so deep that you engaged your email, "read" it, but retained nothing because your conscious awareness was not on the device. The body is on autopilot, and it *loves* being on autopilot because it requires less energy. But being on autopilot is only great if our habits are good for our welfare. If we are unskillful in our affairs and develop poor habits, the autopilot programs run with negative impacts, compounding and deepening as they are repeated.

We do not always recognize the patterns that do not serve us because we have been doing them for so long that we don't think about it or don't question it. Or worse, we justify it even though we know it isn't good for us. Creating healthy, positively compounding habits is the only way you successfully take lifestyle goals and make them accessible. If it is too hard of a fit, the extra effort necessary to maintain it will keep us from actually doing the work to make it a reality.

One way to illustrate how we use our energy related to our tasks is through brain wave states. The brain wave states are consistent throughout genders, ages, and cultures. Our typical active state is called beta, and it's happening right now as you read this—comprehending, communicating, problem-solving, and/or assessing your surroundings. The lower relaxation state is called alpha. The brain waves slow down, and the senses take in less information. Alpha is when you feel like you have been on the go for a while, and then you come to rest. . . and feel yourself get heavy. . . you let out a sigh, maybe your eyes even go unfocused. We relax but lose lots of the details too. Below alpha is theta state, associated with creative flow, meditation, and dreaming. An example of theta is when riding on the highway for a while, and we have a really good idea but can't recall the last couple of miles traveled. The lowest state is delta, the dreamless sleep state. All brain wave states are present at any given time; it's just that one simply predominates, depending on the circumstances. This means that even during active beta state, delta waves are humming somewhere quietly down below our conscious awareness.

Healthy sleep habits that get us into delta wave state are foundational to our well-being. Too often, sleep is overlooked because we view it like shutting down. Instead of thinking of sleep as a shutdown or a reboot, you should view it as an alternate running mode, what I like to call 3R Mode. When delta waves predominate our brains and we go into a dreamless sleep, it allows our bodies to actively enter into a variety of processes that we cannot access in wakeful states. We can broadly categorize these functions as the 3Rs: repairing, refreshing, and recording.

3R Mode allows our bodies' physical internal processes to slow down, specifically our heart rate. The raging rapids of our flowing blood ease into a lazy river, and in the slower current, functions like muscle and organ repair happen easier by not fighting against the stream of a wakeful body. Physical wounds heal faster and kids grow more while asleep. But when you cut your finger or sprain your ankle, it's unlikely your instinct is to go to bed. That's because repairs are only a small part of the functions performed in deep sleep. Most of the internal processes of sleep are for our brains.

In the delta brain wave state, you are dreamless. Being mostly unconscious to the physical world, we do not process much of the sensory data around us and our brains begin to flush out all the neurotoxins that have accumulated throughout the day. Our brains are always giving off a little exhaust as they create thoughts, like a room slowly filling with smoke. Some of these toxins can only be flushed during 3R Mode, the equivalent of opening a window to air out the smoky room. The windows only open in 3R Mode, and the activity of the wakeful brain states keeps the windows locked. If we do not get into the deepest sleep stages and air out, we wake up groggy. We still have fumes. Brain fog and burnout happen when the toxins do not escape because the windows could not be opened.

Each of us has likely experienced a moment where we catch ourselves blankly staring, not retaining anything we are watching, reading, or blindly scrolling through. Then we close our eyes for a moment, and everything resets. Sometimes this is called a micro-sleep or micro-nap, a few seconds or less when delta waves suddenly predominate. That quick flush clears you up enough to say, *I should go to bed* or *I need a cup of coffee*. But regardless of the time of day, the response should always be a moment of rest because that is the only way to enter 3R Mode. In a state of brain fog, we may try to power through, waiting for some inspiration to come out and keep us going, especially in creative endeavors. Many of us have experienced our wheels spinning, going nowhere in such a state. We can't power through the locked windows. We need to open them.

As a species we are sleeping more than ever because the primary function of deep sleep is cataloging our experiences and memories. We need more sleep than our ancestors because we process a significantly wider range of sensory information daily than our predecessors. We have many more muscle memories to dominate the number of tasks that come with modern life filled with technology. We are bombarded daily by information to all of our senses through media, our work, advertisements, education, and personal relationships. A kindergartener may have more social interactions to manage in a school environment than a tribal leader of old.

This information recording process is only available to us in deep sleep. Perhaps you have heard how staying up all night and cramming before a test does not work? The reason is without entering a full sleep cycle filled with 3R Mode, most of that information is lost—it is too much information for too little a cataloging period of time. In fact, if you want to have a better memory, a lifestyle of simplicity creates less for the brain to record each night, less fumes to clear out, less wounds to repair.

What you witness throughout the day will be what you have to catalog at night. We should be mindful of what media and leisure activities we choose to consume and how much of it. I bet you can think of a creepy character that frightened you as a kid, likely from a scary movie, and then haunted your dreams for a while. Consider it cataloged. 3R Mode is the system making what we are experiencing, witnessing, and choosing to focus on literally a part of us. Remember that thoughts only gain momentum if we put energy into them. Choose wisely.

People who struggle with sleep often suffer because they have habits that do not support all three functions of repairing, refreshing, and recording from happening at their best. By creating a sleeping environment that naturally signals the body to enter 3R Mode, we can fall asleep with ease instead of waiting for exhaustion to overcome us. Here are some tips you can try tonight.

- » **Keep it dark**—turn off all blue lights and screens. Keep it quiet. If you are a person who needs the television or noise to fall asleep, try downsizing the amount of ambient light by switching to streaming on a mobile device. Reduce the likelihood of overstimulation or interrupted sleep by selecting something that will turn off automatically once complete, so there is no noise playing throughout the night.
- » **Arrange all your sleeping elements**—pillow, mattress, blankets—to support a straight spine. Find the "Goldilocks Spot"—not too soft, not too hard. Be mindful of your neck; ensure it is in line with the spine and that you can take the deepest breath possible in this position. There is no powering through the pain with sleep; discomfort wakes you up.
- » **Leave a gap of three hours minimum** between eating and sleep to reduce any potential indigestion. Try reducing the sugar and caffeine consumed after lunch, and skip dessert.

You can also try listening to a guided meditation before bed or something that will detach your mind from anything that was bothering you during the day. Get in a little daily exercise to stretch your body and sleep more comfortably. Finish your day seeking a period of time dedicated simply to transitioning to sleep. The disconnected feeling of staring at the TV but not being able to fall asleep happens when the brain and the body are not on the same page. But in these moments, burning off extra energy with some jumping jacks right before bed is not the answer. In fact, the raised heart rate may make it more difficult to fall asleep. Try to work out in the morning, move throughout the day, and allow the body and mind to rest together, peacefully easing into our most restful mode of being.

When we are overtired, it feels as if we are moving through the mud. It is an easy example of how doing the same task with the same expenditure of energy can feel very different. When you are tired, everything is harder, including maintaining your meditation. We can surely think of a time when a bout of crankiness obscured what we meant to do or say. Same goes for when we were hungry. Or had a nasty headache. Or woke up all stiff. By handling the basics of energy management by getting enough quality food and rest, we set our foundation to move through life more alert and ready for adventure.

REFLECTIONS

Do I ease into sleep or do I crash into it?

Have I recently reviewed or refined my sleeping arrangement to fit my body?

Does my mind race while in bed? What do I focus on? Are they the same things that come up during meditation?

Am I getting enough sleep?

What can I make for dinner that would support my sleep habits?

How long after dinner do I go to bed?

What activities can I do, or stop doing, to better support my sleep habits?

Are there any fears that come up at night?

Any denial?

*fall in love with
design,
process,
flow.*

*we are not
an outcome,
product,
result.*

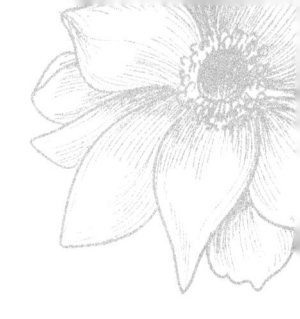

4

EXERCISE

IF WE ARE DOING the spiritual work by cooking our food, practicing meditation, and comfortably resting through full sleep cycles, we may initially feel that we are losing a lot of free time. Maybe you are sleeping more or getting up earlier to practice. Maybe you have to drive a little further to find the groceries that check all the boxes. If you feel a little stretched during these beginning stages, it is good practice to reflect on what you are really giving up and what you are getting back for your new efforts.

Hopefully you are shedding habits and time killers that are not serving you well, while making additional space for your practices to flourish comfortably. If it is still too crammed, keep sifting through the *stuff*. Do not quit. It is okay if you try something new and it fails. That may be a signal that you were on a better track originally, or maybe it sheds light on the reality that you continue to have poor instincts on the matter. We will not learn if we do not experiment and keep paying attention to our choices and their outcomes. That is how our brains work.

Keep refining and working the processes. Keep trying new ideas if the first ones are a bust.

If you need fresh mentors to serve as examples, I think we can agree that you have to be pretty darn wise to be a centenarian, someone who lives to be over one hundred years old. Throughout the world there are "Blue Zones," places that have more centenarians than anywhere else on the planet. Although scattered around the globe in a variety of climates, these communities are made up of mostly farmers and share commonalities in their way of life. The people have an active lifestyle, one that includes daily exercise through physical labors of stretching, pulling, planting, and shoveling, which keeps their bodies limber and flexible. They walk to most places. They chop wood and make things by hand. This type of daily engagement, connecting the mind and body through their work, keeps them young.

Most of us do not live in these conditions, and we may have bad habits from our work life, so we try to compensate for them with fitness workouts. We sit all day, so we go for a run. We do not participate in physical labor, so we go lift barbells after work. There is nothing wrong with this, and it is obviously better than doing nothing. But our bodies have not biologically changed very much since ancient times, and this is not how our ancestors lived. They were nomads and traversed difficult terrains during all seasons. We may not even go outside if it's too cold or rainy. They walked for hours a day, sifting through bushes and bending to check grasses and tracks.

We may go all day without touching the floor, unless we drop something. And we can go on and on about how sedentary we are becoming, especially when compared with previous generations.

Conscious daily movements can fit into two categories: fitness and exercise. While for some of us these may be the same activities, for others they are separate practices worthy of distinction. There is no one-size-fits-all, and there are plenty of people without the need or interest in fitness who are living healthy lives.

The idea of "fitness" refers to a specific physical activity performed for our bodies for a definite purpose. Whether it's losing a few extra pounds, wanting to bench-press more than our body weight, getting six-pack abs, or building the stamina to athletically compete, daily life is unlikely to include enough activity for you to become this fit, and you must engage in fitness workouts to achieve your goals. Fitness is similar to meditation practice in that it requires us to stop all of our other activities and focus completely on the present moment. How much time you dedicate to fitness is an individual question, but a common recommendation for fitness workouts is a minimum of three days a week, with the aim of getting into a detoxifying, full-body sweat during those sessions.

Exercise is a broader category of daily movements through active lifestyle and wellness practices, including simple things like walking after dinner, doing yoga or tai chi, biking your errands instead of driving, and engaging in active outdoor hobbies. It may not always require getting sweaty, and the positive results may be less visual or obvious when compared to fitness routines.

Exercise is a form of preventative medicine, keeping our systems working with efficiency to maintain homeostasis. When we are well, we have stamina, concentration, and feel loose and relaxed. When we focus on keeping our bodies running clean and efficiently, we support good circulation, joint health, proper posture, a strong heart, appropriate nervous system reactivity, and comfortable, calm breathing. Exercise cleans out the system, and it's more like a daily dusting to keep things fresh, rather than a deep spring cleaning.

Exercise within your spectrum, even if fitness feels unrealistic right now. Learn from the "Blue Zones" example. In contrast to fitness, exercise does not adhere to a "no pain, no gain" mentality but is more about keeping a regular schedule of daily movement, naturally integrated into your lifestyle. Exercise is an opportunity for self-love, an integration of mind and body.

However we choose to move each day, exercise is a practice for awakening because it gives us a direct line into understanding karma. Karma is another loaded word these days. A common misunderstanding of karma is an "eye for an eye," an equal punishment for a wrongdoing. But karma is not a source of punishment or a great equalizer. Another misconception of karma is "if you do good things, good things will happen to you." While this can be true, it is not that karma is rewarding anyone. These personifications of karma acting like a parent to keep things fair confuse the nature of what we are talking about. Karma is an unbiased force, not a moral compass.

Part of the confusion stems from viewing karma as a result, when karma is really the action. Our actions, how and where we put our energy, will determine our outcomes. You gain momentum from each decision. Karma pushes energy indiscriminately, with the potential to lean toward proper or poor habits, depending on what we reinforce through our behavior. Karma does not discern what is best for you or how to alter the course; it simply moves forward. We must be skillful to successfully work with karma so that we do not struggle against it.

Addictions are examples of unskillfully working with karma. Numerous poor decisions build upon each other, making it harder and harder to break the bad habit that has formed. It may begin innocently, but it gets reinforced by repeating the same actions, going to the same places, or spending time with the same people. There is a recurrence of events that continues to gain momentum, making the abusive habit harder to stop.

For example, maybe it's after the third drink that things go south. It's not just one decision, that last drink. Rather, it is the ongoing culmination of decisions and familiar poor habits—going to the bar, seeing the usual crowd, sipping that first drink, then a second—compounding upon each other. When it is time to pump the brakes on that third drink, there is a whole night's worth of momentum to upend. Maybe we are having a good time and convince ourselves we can handle one more drink. Or maybe we are having a poor time and rationalize one more drink to pick things up. With all that energy in motion, particularly in a situation where we are unskillful, it is unlikely we can bargain our way out of the final behavior that leads to negative consequences.

If you are unskillful 100 times, you may need to be skillful in the same situation 101 times to correct it. Sometimes it really is that straightforward. Other times it may require a set of completely new habits to counter the one we wish to eliminate. Each moment is interconnected by each decision, each action, one building upon the next. That's karma: the force that keeps moving us, building and destroying, keeping all of these individual pieces linked together, like the unbiased current that connects the water to make a river.

When we say that a person has good karma, it isn't magic, luck, or mystical power. It's not the karma itself that we are picking up on but the steadiness and confidence this individual has cultivated over time by making the right decisions. When you work well with karma, you trust your instincts more. We stay present, notice when we take the proper actions, and repeat them. We must be equally honest and acknowledge when we are unskillful, correcting our behaviors when necessary.

EXERCISE

Exercise and fitness are great practices for learning to work with karma. The physical sensations of working your body can provide more immediate feedback than working with karma on emotional levels. Many yoga traditions have students practice only one sequence of postures, at the same time each day, to create a baseline experience to begin working with karma. Despite repeating the same exact motions day after day, students notice the range of unique feelings that come up within each practice session. Utilizing meditation and physical practices as daily check-in points helps us to notice the differences of each day and which of yesterday's choices are supporting or hindering us now.

If you stay disciplined, chances are the practices will get easier with time, a sign of working well with karma. But you may not have the same energy level each day, and that could relate more to your eating and sleeping habits than your discipline about daily movements. Energy levels are directly linked to each other by how well we sleep, the quality of what we eat, and how well we handle our physical tasks. A bad diet will likely override any gains we make through exercise, and poor sleep will always make things worse. By relating our daily habits to each other, we step out of compartmentalizing our lives and start living as a whole being, growing in awareness of how each of our decisions are interconnected to one another.

The most important element of working with karma is to keep noticing, without judging ourselves. If you witness something you do not like, you have the ability to make a different choice next time. If we see a pattern that is gaining momentum without serving us well, we can pump the brakes. By taking a step back and just noticing, we make a little space to see ourselves objectively, and we are less likely to react impulsively or repeat the same mistakes.

Undoing bad habits takes time. There is a gap between the moment that you notice something you want to change and having the ability to successfully change it. We usually have to slow the momentum of the bad habit before we can change direction. Like a speeding car, if we do not slow down first, we may flip over or spiral out of control when we abruptly try to change directions. Be patient.

Bringing our whole being to our daily practices of cooking, sleeping, exercise, and meditation may feel burdensome at first and seemingly impossible to fit into our schedules. By identifying and shedding the poor habits we notice, we can make the necessary space to support these integral practices. When encountering extra spaciousness, allow the practices to echo in the emptiness instead of immediately filling in these gaps with something new. As you learn to work with karma by creating habits that serve you well and sticking to them, you'll begin to notice additional resources offered in each moment. We can drift along with karma, steady in ourselves, trusting enough to look up and enjoy the stars as we comfortably float on life's currents.

REFLECTIONS

Am I happy with my body?

What is enough exercise for me to feel well?

Am I moving enough today, or do I feel tight?

What am I doing to offset physical habits, such as lots of sitting, computer hunch, or working more with one hand?

Do I have any habits that conflict with each other?

Is there anything I can do to increase my love for my body?

Do I treat my body and mind as separate? Does my body suffer because of it?

Has it been a while since I've done something kind for my body or mind?

How do you harness the power of the universe in a single moment?

With a flower.
Or a stone.
A few leaves.
A seasonally inspired infusion.
A peaceful atmosphere
to hear the rain.

Space to simply be.
Space to acknowledge how small we are
compared to how big we feel.
Space to laugh at ourselves
and forgive ourselves.

To say,
I am here now,
despite my errors.

Space to turn it all around.

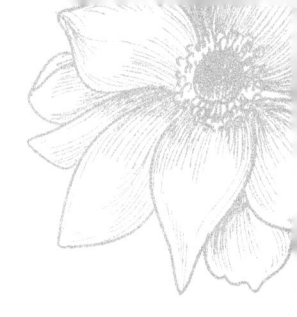

5

MEDITATION

MEDITATION PRACTICE IS THE key to breaking through from a healthy life to an awakened one. If we practice being honest, eating well, sleeping well, and exercising daily, we will feel better and have more energy. But what to do with this newfound energy? We need to focus so it does not give us more power to be destructive or foolishly pursue desires that do not serve us. Let us now dig deeper into the definition of meditation.

Meditation is the state of being fully aware in the present moment without judgment. This is my personal working definition of meditation, an attempt at the ineffable, primarily influenced by Chögyam Trungpa Rinpoche. Let's break it down together.

Meditation is a state of being, <u>not</u> an action. We don't meditate. There is no "meditating." We sit on cushions and *formally practice entering* the *state of meditation*. Using meditation as a verb is like saying that you are "happying" when you enjoy a nice meal with your friends.

Tasting delicious food, laughing, and socializing create the conditions for happiness to naturally arise—you don't try to happy, it just *happens* when you are enjoying yourself. In meditation practice, the conditions can be sitting in silence, engaging in a certain breathing pattern, focusing our awareness, when meditation naturally arises (or at least, we are giving ourselves the best, distraction-free chance to do so). Each awakening tradition has its own set of techniques to facilitate entering the state of meditation. The best practice technique is the one you are willing to continue practicing.

Meditation is being fully aware. To be fully aware is to experience life with honesty and clarity, both on the emotional level and through our senses. Our brains are calculating probabilities and trying to anticipate our environment through the information collected by the senses. Most of these systems are run by autonomic systems and operate outside of our conscious control. Our conscious awareness, our attention, is what we can control. Yet we are usually very scattered with this awareness. Meditation practice techniques show us how to focus our energy and how to keep our attention consciously on our actions. When we act with mindfulness, our actions are intentional. With focused, open awareness, we reduce our chances of causing accidental harm or misinterpreting our surroundings, making it easier to maintain harmony with those around us.

Meditation is in the present moment. Many of us spend too much time ping-ponging between thoughts about the past and dreams about the future. We work at our jobs and only half of our brain is doing the grind. The other half is off planning our next holiday, or worrying about credit card debt, or replaying that silly thing we said to a person we admire, or thinking about dinner. These thoughts are distractions occupying our attention, keeping us away from the here and now. They also block our view from seeing all the potential possibilities at our disposal in a given moment. To be present is to deal with what is directly in front of us, not to be mentally somewhere else. Even when these mental tasks seem productive, we can often avoid pitfalls by focusing our full effort in the present. That will give us our best likelihood of success in the future.

Meditation is without judgment. We are clouded by our own thoughts, biases, and judgments as our brains are running all the probabilities, trying to predict the next moment. For example, we often do not listen to what others are saying because we are thinking of what we are going to say next, especially in an argument. To accurately perceive things precisely as they are, we need to listen. Being fully aware often feels slowed down, as we take in data through the senses and absorb the details before reacting. We do not suddenly act like sloths, but we give our brains an extra moment to process everything before running the response sequence. This allows us to see things as they are, not as the first thing that popped into our minds or as we wish them to be.

With practice, we can maintain openness in the face of challenging emotions, on and off the cushion.

The process of awakening helps the practitioner shed all the *stuff* that is not theirs and authentically own the rest. We shed false expectations, worries, the karma of past mistakes, fears, and the thoughts that keep us from being our best. These are the judgments distorting our perspective—another form of rose-colored glasses—that keep us from seeing things clearly. We also need to own our decisions and accept all the things that made us the way we are now. We own our actions; we shed our thoughts. We are not our thoughts. When we inappropriately over identify with our thoughts and solidify our sense of individual self, we enter protection-mode for selfish interests and lose sight of the fact that we are part of something much bigger. Problems come when solidifying our identity creates not only a sense of *self* but, more detrimentally, a sense of *others*.

Awakening does not ask you to pretend to enjoy all things equally or give up the things you love. We will always have preferences. But it does require us to correct the moments when we allow preferred desires to cloud our judgment and justify doing the selfish, wrong actions. As you sit in silence, no one can hear you or hurt you as you work your *stuff*. Meditation practice is an opportunity to silently let go of these judgments and open your heart.

Now, let us dispel some common misconceptions about meditation and its practice.

Meditation is not shutting off our brain or stopping our thoughts. This is a common misconception. Your brain *is* a thought machine, running statistical probabilities at a rate faster than any other known organ or machine on Earth, while simultaneously coordinating electrical pulses to orchestrate movement of the body based on signals from the outside world obtained by the senses, *and additionally* having conscious mental thoughts in relationship to, and independent of, those functions. And that's just you walking on the sidewalk, smelling pizza, and thinking about lunch. We only exert a limited amount of control through our conscious awareness. We cannot stop our thoughts. Meditation practice does not seek the impossible of shutting down the brain but instead gives us a viewpoint to recognize our thought patterns and how we react to them.

When we begin practicing, we may feel like our minds are televisions flicking through the channels, and we do not have control of the remote. But with training, we can sharpen our focus to experience fewer channels and less inner button-pushing. During practice we continue focusing on a single channel, one that plays the same show on repeat: the breath. We come back to this channel whenever we find ourselves mentally scrolling again. Distractions change the channel. . . a stomach grumble. . . hmm, what is for lunch? Tune back into the breath. Discomfort changes the channel. . . a foot is falling asleep. . . tune back in again. This tuning in is not forceful. It should feel light, as easy as clicking the button. If we notice our minds scrolling like crazy, it's okay. That was today's program. What did you learn? No matter the experience the mind remains turned on. The question is: Are we tuned in?

Meditation is <u>not</u> fantasizing or imagining. Sitting around and daydreaming is not meditation. Focusing on anything outside of the practice while the timer is running is not being present (*even great ideas for the book you want to write about awakening!*). Do not worry that these ideas will not return to you. We are practicing entering the fertile, creative state of meditation so that this awareness is more readily accessible to us in the opportune moments when we really need it.

During practice, just practice. Focus your awareness and reserve being creative for afterwards. To be blunt, if we are thinking about anything other than following the breath (or other object of focus), then we are in fantasy land. Even when a great idea appears, let it go. It will come back.

When practicing meditation, we do <u>not</u> have goals. There are plenty of self-help books out there on how to meditate for maximum results, but no genuine spiritual practice has such metrics. Meditation practice is spiritual. To make it anything less is to miss out on its greatest opportunities. Practicing with a proper teacher can help students continue to reach their potential. Someone with more experience can aid us with our hang-ups about progress or doing it right. A good teacher can help us identify our inner disruptions, especially someone who knows us well and is familiar with our practice technique. A spiritual friend can help us interpret our experience without allowing us to get trapped by our minds during times of trial. Even when we have a road map for what is expected ahead, each of us will have a unique experience. Begin from wherever you are, and do not compare yourself. Seeking results at speed does not make them come faster. Simply put, the only goal we have is to complete each practice successfully and be stalwart enough to do it again... and again... and again...

Meditation practice is about openness, not happiness. Although increased happiness is a common side effect! If we could replace "I just want to be happy" with "I want to feel open," we could work ourselves closer to that happiness that seems so elusive. But let us be clear: meditation is not a bliss state, it is an honest one. In fact, many beginners walk away from the practice because they are searching for a bliss state, an altered state, like being high on drugs but without the substances. Whatever the technique, meditation practice is tough in the beginning, just like the learning curve of any new skill. In the world of social media, meditation is often paraded around as a cure-all or the big secret to happiness—but there is no magic, and nothing comes without the exertion. However, when we do the work and open ourselves, meditation offers us greater possibilities, which usually leads to greater joy.

Beauty and abundance surround us, but we are just too picky about our ideas of happiness. We narrowly seek out situations and people to serve our desired version of things, and we miss a lot of opportunities because of this tunnel vision. Too many of us go into hiding during moments of boredom or discomfort, waiting around for the next highly stimulating, desire-fulfilling moment to arrive. You may waste a lot of time hanging around and seeking desire, instead of enjoying each moment for all it is worth.

In yoga, we do hear about amazing teachers that enter the awakened state of *samadhi* and cry blissful tears. But they come down from this spiritual "high" because it is only a side effect of meditation, not the practice itself. The bliss ends, but the wisdom does not. It's been said, "After the ecstasy comes the laundry," and we must continue to be present after such an experience and not get attached to it. Seeking these spiritual highs is a form of spiritual materialism, and it only distracts us from being open to all experiences. It is not the state of meditation itself that makes us happy, it is the openness to see the beauty and the mystery of our lives that is so blissfully overwhelming.

Establishing a formal meditation practice will give you a mental baseline to notice where the mind goes when it wanders. That's where your attention is going when it ditches the present moment. We have to be very conscious and honest about what our feelings are and how we are working with them. These thoughts keep replaying in our nervous systems, whether we admit it or not. When we maintain our practices for a balanced state of being, we stay open to possibilities, see things as they are, and reduce the chances of miscalculating from our expectations or judgments. If life is going to unexpectedly push us, it is better that we have both feet comfortably well-grounded than to tempt fate on one foot.

Practice every day, even if only for a few minutes in the beginning. Consistency is more important than the length of each session. Five minutes a day, every day, is better than an hour only on weekends. When you find a practice that works, try to stick with it. You may get overexcited and collect as many techniques as possible because *variety is the spice of life!* It is wonderful to diversify experiences in order to home in on what really supports you. But at some point, you need to buckle down with a singular method. The real challenge is to dedicate oneself to the same technique every day and notice how no two sessions are the same. Those insights are only available through proper repetition. Explore, have fun, and keep coming back to one practice that consistently nourishes you with a sense of calm and introspection. That is likely the best practice for you.

Once we can feel the difference between meditation and operating unskillfully, we take our formal practice off of the cushion and into our everyday experience: noticing, slowing down, seeing our patterns, seeing all options, not becoming attached to outcomes or certain directions, taking each present moment as it is and working with what is right in front of us. Identifying the areas in your life that are not serving you well is vital for spiritual growth. By quieting our minds and listening with our whole being, answers and opportunities can show themselves without the need for such fervent seeking.

Practicing meditation by sitting in silence and noticing where the mind goes is the easiest, cost-nothing, can-do-it-anywhere type of practice to see exactly where we need to put our energy to become more balanced, relaxed, and open to our world. For me, it was the difference between doing a bunch of random things for my health and beginning to genuinely understand the connection between my actions and my feelings. It is an ongoing investigation, and all insights are only temporary in a world of ever-changing conditions. Everything is impermanent: the good times and the bad. The next moment is already on your doorstep. Just keep practicing.

REFLECTIONS

Am I practicing meditation enough?

Am I getting to a peaceful place in my practice? How long does it last?

What thoughts continuously surface during my practice?

Do I find myself in the present moment when I practice?

Do I find myself in the past or the future? Why?

Is my formal practice reflecting in my life off the cushion?

What is the difference between peace and relaxation?

Can I cultivate joy just sitting in an empty room?

Can I bring this joy into every moment?

Each of us walks the path alone.
Loneliness is part of the human condition.
The trick is to be friends with yourself,
stay in good company.
Then everyone you meet joins a wonderful party.

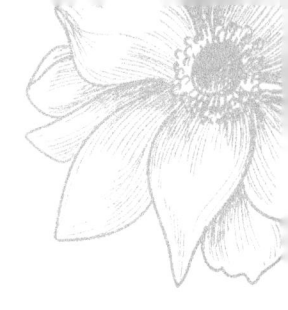

6

CURIOSITY

TO CONTINUE OUR DISCUSSION on awakening, we have to gain a richer understanding of the body-mind connections that operate outside of our conscious control. The autonomic nervous system maintains vital functions of the internal organs and digestive tract, including our heartbeat, breathing, and saliva production, helping us maintain homeostasis for a variety of inner systems. It contains three parts, but this discussion will focus on the two interconnected wings.

The sympathetic wing is the "fight-or-flight" response that monitors hunger, gauges excitement, and raises our heart rate to pump blood to the sensory systems, keeping us wary of danger. When triggered, it shifts your body into an alternate survival mode that includes physical changes. Our pupils dilate to take in more detailed surroundings, our blood thickens for faster healing if injured, and our breath shortens to pump oxygen to our limbs. The body literally prepares to fight a death match or escape as fast as possible if outmatched. Sympathetic engagement is not designed as a long-term state of being, but a short and powerful shift to do what is necessary to triumph or flee. Once safe, the fight-or-flight response disengages, and the opposite side, the parasympathetic wing, engages to restore us to equilibrium.

Your parasympathetic wing is the anatomical mind-body connection that induces resting, digestion, and healing, including relaxed feelings after eating and "yoga glow" after a deep practice. The functions of the parasympathetic wing are only available to us when we feel safe and comfortable.

The two wings are interconnected; as one side engages, the other disengages. Our natural state is one of balance between the two sides, with the parasympathetic wing primarily engaged to maintain homeostasis, and the fight-or-flight response ready to activate at any sign of trouble, making for an equilibrium state that is inherently relaxed, yet alert. Our senses transmit the information necessary to understand our environment and choose which side of the system to engage.

Because it is imperative to your survival to accurately predict danger, your mind has a negativity bias to focus on dangerous cues more than on rewards. After all, one misjudgment of danger and we could be dead! Our brains are even willing to misinterpret the signal and send us the most dangerous possibility in the name of survival. If you have ever mistaken a coat rack for an intruder, that is your negativity bias working to keep you safe.

Today, most of us do not face the kinds of mortal perils of our ancestors, who were fearful of physical attacks from predators or rival tribes, but our sympathetic wing is still triggered regularly by stressful social situations and sensory overstimulation. The ugly reality is that the system does not distinguish between mortal peril, public embarrassment, pressure from work, an off-putting comment from a relative, or bad hair days: the engagement of the sympathetic wing is the same survival cascade, looking to fight or flee from whatever negative cue triggered the system. It treats all bad feelings, whether emotional or physical, as danger.

The sympathetic wing is also triggered by surprises, including phones ringing, alerts vibrating, and emails buzzing all day and night. As we are the first generations to live with these technologies, the impact it's truly had on us is not simple to quantify. The daily barrage of signals that our senses are asked to digest is unprecedented. The relentless unpredictability of the next message keeps our minds and senses perpetually engaged, often sparking the fight-or-flight response inappropriately. It is becoming increasingly clear that constant overstimulation of the sympathetic wing has negative health consequences, leading to imbalances in the body caused by excessive excretion of stress hormones. An overactive fight-or-flight response disgruntles our nervous systems and breaks down immunity, making the way for illness.

Many of us need to take additional measures to rebalance our ancient biology with our changing modern environment. We need to set clear boundaries so that we give our nervous system the ability to reset properly. You may not be in a position to simply unplug and immediately change your way of living, but you can introduce activities that intentionally diffuse the feeling of overwhelm. The good news is that we have already discussed ways to disengage ourselves into a parasympathetic healing state, through meditation practice, exercise, quality sleep, and a nutrient-rich diet.

Additionally, a curious attitude is a great equalizer for negativity bias because it lets us approach uncertainty with engagement instead of fear. A learning brain is a happy brain, even when we make mistakes and acquire hard lessons. In those moments, we need to focus on the good while looking at the results in earnest and stay open to new challenges instead of closing down. The more we can focus on the positive, without denying the negative, the less power we give unfortunate circumstances when they come upon us unexpectedly.

Find an activity or hobby that you can treat as your curiosity practice, something that stimulates all three of the following happiness brain chemicals. *Dopamine* is one of our powerful neurotransmitters, released when we are motivated or excited. Our practice should keep us continuously engaged, building upon skills we are learning and encouraging progress. *Oxytocin* is the relationship neurotransmitter, released during social bonding, particularly when we spend time with people we care about, do something good for someone else, or receive something pleasant. Once we have a proficiency in our craft, our curiosity practice should be something we can share with others, even if we practice it alone. *Serotonin* is the neurotransmitter released when we feel superior or do something successfully and are praised for it, but it also regulates mood and memory. It's where we get that extra boost from a feeling of victory, and our practice should include milestones we can achieve without getting lost in our ego. When we practice something that brings us pleasure, has ongoing milestones, and is something that we can share and teach to others, we give ourselves the prospect of finding happiness without seeking it.

Your curiosity practice can be something with lofty, long-term goals, such as finding a faraway land to visit, saving up for the trip, and learning the language. Or when seeing something we would like to buy, we can learn the skills to create it ourselves, like knitting a scarf or building a birdhouse. Pick up a musical instrument or art form and study it deeply. Add something to your life that helps you relate directly to your experience, engages your senses, and asks you to be present when doing it. If there is little space in your life for new activities, get creative about mixing awakening practices together. Perhaps you are taking a daily walk in a park and can learn what types of plants reside there. Find new recipes as you continue to take control over all your meals. Pick a difficult yoga posture and dedicate some practices specifically to the poses that will help you get into that posture. Whenever possible, include doing this practice in nature because the outdoors is a great catalyst for all three happiness chemicals.

Whatever activity you choose for your practice, it must be active, not passive. We all need occasional breaks to shut down sometimes, but the purpose of this practice is to engage our minds in unique ways. It should not be a form of escapism. Anything in which we are passive spectators like watching movies (generally any entertainment consumption) will not qualify.

Amidst the conveniences of our modern world, we can thrive so well without experiencing true discomfort that we create problems out of boredom or inappropriately high expectations. Our appreciation of good circumstances deteriorates under the grind of other emotions like jealousy, anger, or apathy. The first symptoms are often restlessness, feeling stuck in a rut, and/or spending too much time scrolling the web. If we are in tune enough to feel deterioration coming on, we can reach for our curiosity practice to give us a boost of novelty and snap us out of it.

Curiosity practice is another opportunity to express meditation in your actions. It doesn't necessarily have to be something that is productive outside of keeping you spiritually engaged. In the grand scheme of things, maybe it is not so important to be able to do a handstand, but maybe trying to do a handstand is the practice that keeps us from engaging in the poor habits we are trying to correct. Maintaining focus on the process and not on the end results can be a lifelong practice. Make a little progress daily. Keep a journal. Reflect on your journey. Simplify your life so you can handle your responsibilities and still have time to focus on things you truly relish. When engaging in activities we enjoy with people we love, it becomes more obvious how little we really need to be happy.

REFLECTIONS

What have I learned lately?

What do I participate in that brings me joy and peace?

Have I done anything lately that really excites me?

Am I repeating my mistakes or am I learning from them?

When I relax, am I refreshing myself or numbing out?

CURIOSITY

Am I using my practice to become a better communicator?

What changes have I made to alter a poor habit?

How can I express myself without having to say anything?

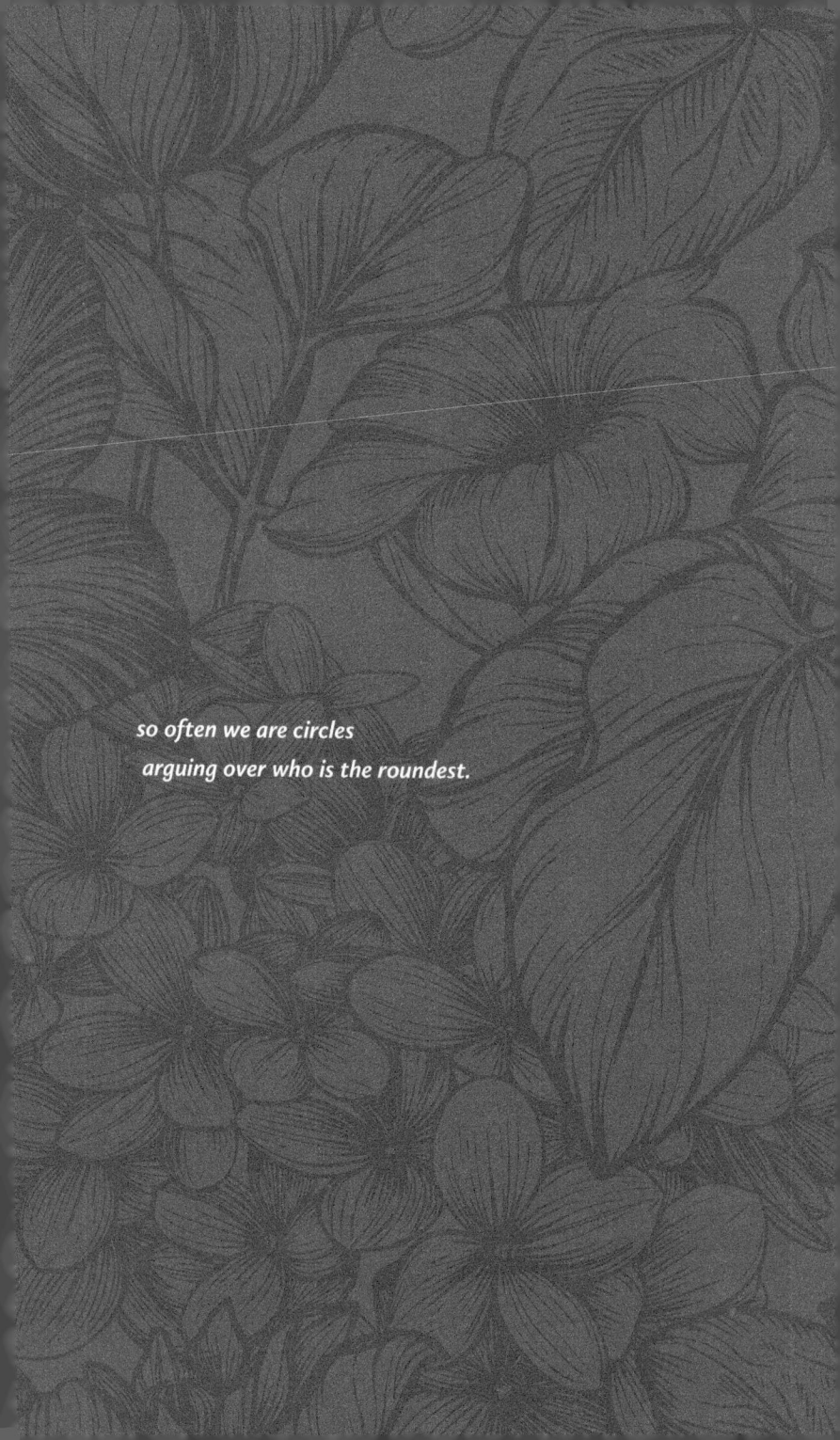

so often we are circles
  arguing over who is the roundest.

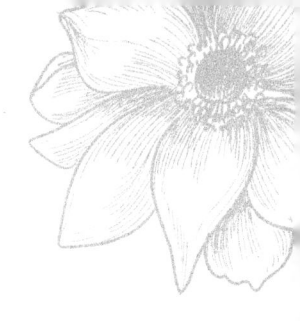

7

RELATIONSHIPS

IN MANY AWAKENING TRADITIONS, seekers leave home and go into seclusion, becoming hermits in the wilderness. Disconnected from daily challenges and social distractions, nature becomes the primary teacher. They can focus exclusively on their inner being, undisturbed by others. But in interdependent modern life, few of us can drop all our responsibilities and withdraw into the woods. Rest assured it is not necessary to disappear from society to become awakened. Spirituality is not somewhere *out there*, it is within us, regardless of where we stand on the planet. If we really want liberation from our woes, we need to do the work right where we are, where it matters most.

The daily grind likely repeats undesirable challenges. You may notice patterns consuming large amounts of mental space because you cannot distance yourself from them. When we're stuck in a loop that we cannot seem to escape, friction keeps increasing until we give it space to stop rubbing us the wrong way. Self-care practices can help you gain the necessary space to end the friction and come back refreshed. Hopefully all the keys we have discussed thus far qualify as self-care, but you may require additional outlets to disconnect far enough and long enough to feel revitalized. Practices can be as simple as alone time with the door shut, going for a long walk, spending extended time in nature, or digging into a book. Even if we indulge in pleasures for a while, self-care is not a selfish act if practiced responsibly. Be mindful of binging in ways that ignore responsibilities or lose sight of the needs of those around us. Self-care is doing what is necessary for your health, to maintain inner balance and strength. When it is time to reconnect, ask yourself if you are now ready to handle the situation you were distancing yourself from. If the answer is yes, that is a good practice. When we *feel* good, we are more likely to *do* good.

Self-care offers us an opportunity to pay special attention to our senses. Eastern philosophies teach that we have six senses. The first four are the familiar seeing, hearing, smelling, and tasting. The fifth extends the sense of touch to the feeling body, including skin and physical sensations like getting the chills, pangs of hunger, pins and needles from a foot falling asleep, or stiffness in the muscles. The sixth sense is the mind, the interpreter for the other senses. You may hear or feel your stomach grumble, but the mind tells you to eat. It translates sensations and signals into language that brings information into our conscious awareness, in a way we can understand. Your ears hear the siren, the mind tells you danger. You eat a delicious fruit, and the mind relates the taste with vitamins. A good self-care practice reduces distractions, leaving room to focus on interconnected sensory pathways. Like our curiosity practice, self-care is meditation in action, and our practice should include simple pleasures to synchronize the senses and our mind-body connections.

We have explored how negativity bias tricks us, and it is understandable how senses are similarly vulnerable to deception. Many of our primary brain functions are for translating our world, and there is potential for getting scrambled. A cookie can lie to our brain that it is healthy because we are eating a high concentration of sugar, which it usually equates with fruits filled with vitamins. It is easy to pig out on sweets because our brains are not used to so much sugar, and the autonomic processes are tricked into thinking we have found a new superfruit. . . until satiety catches up and realizes it is all sugar and no vitamins, but we have probably already overindulged before that return signal tells us to stop. Then the body tries to dump off the excess sugar, causing the characteristic sugar rush and crash in kids and catnap in adults. There are many products in our modern world that intentionally manipulate our senses, and generally speaking, they are not good for us.

You are more likely to misinterpret your surroundings when overstimulated or in an environment that triggers your fight-or-flight response. Many of these environments are part of everyday life, as half of us are currently living in urban settings. We are forced to filter through overcrowded commutes as transportation moves us at unnatural speeds. Our civilized world is tough on our senses, not to mention all the advertisements trying to nab our attention as we simply change locations. Many of us have responded to the overwhelm by donning puffy coats, headphones, and big sunglasses, to create a buffer between us and the overload. While these are workable coping strategies, one of our best counterbalances is consciously constructing a space in our homes where we can decompress and practice self-care.

Create a quiet, private space reserved for resetting yourself, meditation practice, contemplation, and emotional unloading (screaming, crying, and crazy laughing included). Design a nucleus for awakening, a personal sanctuary for regaining meditation. Distinct from thinking of our "happy place," which probably has a lot of pleasurable, stimulating experiences attached to it, this is where we come to get a meditation baseline and includes only the essentials.

When customizing your sanctuary, take all six senses into account, offering an environment where each can relax. Try expressions through atmosphere instead of material things. Use natural light and any window views to add ambiance without more objects. Reserve a pleasant scent for this space to give your body a cue that it is time to practice or unwind. Be mindful of too many decorations, for often a cluttered space reflects a cluttered mind. It often requires removing items before the sanctuary feels open *and* contemplative. This may serve as a great window into what *stuff* no longer has a place. It can take time before settling into a comfortable form, and the design process is a practice too, as our outer world begins to mirror our inner world more accurately.

Once the sanctuary design is successfully supporting your meditation, examine other environments you inhabit and apply your new design principles (while being extra mindful of everyone's feelings when approaching shared spaces). Rework each area to reflect the calm now available in your sanctuary. Clean the closet, cabinets, pantry, and make each revision a creative expression that brings organization and delight. Review possessions and sort them into categories of essential, used once in a while, and ready to be let go. Acknowledge the usage rate of your belongings and purge unnecessary items through selling, gifting, donating, or recycling. Practice gratitude for each item and handle its removal with respect. Do not dump stuff on other people or immediately run out to replace possessions with new purchases. Take it slow, leave time to adjust, and evolve organically. Keep incorporating more sustainable options in each adaptation. Can you create a space that induces meditation and leaves no material imprint on the world?

As you reduce your material imprint to a more manageable level, a common bonus is gaining more free time. Decluttering can lead to fewer chores, leaving us to focus on what we enjoy as a social species: our relationships with others.

Each of us possess *mirror neurons*, a biological tool that helps us physically experience each other's moods. They allow us to pick up on emotions before a person speaks, through body language, nonverbal sounds, posture, and facial expressions. When we engage positively with each other, full of smiles and laughter, we can boost our happy chemicals even when doing the simplest things, thanks to our mirror neurons. Nothing can beat the natural resilience and joy that we muster from being around the ones we love. Treasuring the days spent together and fortifying each other with good memories is one of the best supports you can offer. Practicing self-care with loved ones will have compounding effects. Happy feelings are literally contagious.

Mirror neurons are quite the superpower, and like all powers, they have a dark potential. Our connections are a two-way street and they can also reflect negativity. You are likely familiar with someone who walks with a heavy cloud around them, making us want to leave when they enter. When someone yells at you, the fight-or-flight response is triggered, and you want to yell back. These are the important moments to slow down and ensure we respond from a state of meditation. Mirror neurons reflect, but they do not have the power to act. Difficult conversations can turn into a neural standoff, and you can de-escalate aggression by maintaining a positive, peaceful state of mind in the face of the disgruntled. We must be attentive to our feelings so we do not amplify a feedback loop, especially when engaging with those who do not bring out the best in us.

There is an old yogic joke that if you think you have reached enlightenment, go spend the weekend with your parents. While we may love and gather great strength from our closest relatives, those who know you the best also usually know how to push your buttons. These interactions can shine a light into places where we still have attachments.

We are each experiencing new things that are altering our perceptions. In the same way that we do not want to be held to the person we used to be, we must leave space for relationships to change and grow too. We should remember that everyone is not on the same spiritual journey that we are on, and we should not take it personally when others fail to match our kindness or openness.

Even with our toughest relationships, we can operate from our cultivated place of honesty. Acknowledge when someone is trying to take from you in a way that makes you uncomfortable. Honoring those feelings in the moment can keep things clear before they have an opportunity to deteriorate. Maintain personal boundaries where necessary. You cannot always get away from relationships that you do not like, but you can choose how you interact in those relationships. We are not responsible for the feelings of others, but we are responsible for our actions. No one should have to endure abuse, but be wary of prematurely labeling people as toxic. We are all suffering in our own way, we all wish for relief, but too often we are unsure of how or where to find it. We cannot put up a wall or shun those who may bring us down. We cannot bulldoze through life in a shielded bubble of positivity. To endure, we must have empathy for each other through the good times and the bad.

Remember this equation. I first heard it from renowned meditation teacher Shinzen Young, in *The Science of Enlightenment* lectures:

Suffering = Pain x Resistance

Regardless of who you are or what resources are available, pain hurts. Pain is a signal that we are not proceeding correctly. It isn't a bad thing; often it's the warning that we need. When we correct the behavior, the pain stops. But when we resist getting the message, we open ourselves up to further suffering. When we take the pain and multiply it with our emotions, desires, or expectations, we suffer long beyond the pain itself. A lot of resistance comes from our *stuff*. We are the only ones who can create a spacious life for ourselves, to maintain our meditation regardless of the challenges we are facing. Life naturally has ups and downs, but the question is, can you stay open-minded regardless of the conditions? Or do you resist things that ask you to step up or out of your comfort zone?

How we act in our relationships is a daily indicator of how often we are operating from a state of meditation. When we come into peace with ourselves, we act mindfully and with awareness to our surroundings. We avoid many potentials for emotional fallout because we are more sensitive to them. By practicing self-care and honoring our feelings, it gets easier to act with authenticity. You gain an inner comfort, some extra space from not putting on airs, and you do not take it so personally when met with the unflattering or obnoxious. Our mirror neurons will still get triggered, but nothing sticks because we know those feelings do not belong to us.

We control our actions in each of our relationships regardless of the conditions. We always have that extra moment, a deep breath, and the executive brain function, to not simply react but consciously reset our meditation before proceeding. Take care of yourself so you can better take care of the world around you, creating a feedback loop of support. Be the positive light that emblazes a thousand additional candles without sacrificing its own flame.

REFLECTIONS

How am I managing my relationships? Am I antisocial?

Does my self-care support my ongoing health or does it just feel good for a while?

What is my relationship like with technology?

What's my average daily screen time?

Have I spent any time in the sun or in nature lately?

RELATIONSHIPS

Am I living a sustainable life?

Are there areas I can waste less?

Am I living in harmony with the environment?

What can I do in my work environment to be more tolerant of rudeness?

Where does my resistance come from?

Does it keep me from being of service?

Will the decisions made today not only matter today but 300 years from now?

Am I sending storms into our future or cultivating the soil?

*The distinction between
strength and power
is subtle,
yet
the misunderstanding of this difference
leads to great destruction.*

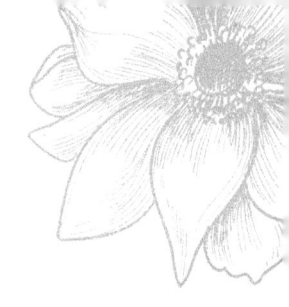

8

RESPONSIBILITY

Operating from meditation allows us to have ease within ourselves, but it does not mean that life becomes easy. To the contrary, life often gets more difficult for a period after beginning an awakening practice. Our cultivated awareness takes in more details. You may feel as if you have superpowers with your fresh sensitivity, but you may also feel raw and exposed by your newfound awareness. It may be tough to step up when we feel weak and vulnerable from our own healing process. Take extra time and do the work correctly. Our first responsibility is to keep ourselves healthy and strong enough to meet our other duties.

Health and stability extend beyond our mind and bodies to include our social bonds, finances, functionality of our possessions, preparedness for emergencies, and more. No matter how robust we are physically, we will die without water in a few days. We need food, warmth, and shelter to sustain ourselves (add basic wilderness skills to curiosity practices if they are not already acquired). If we drive to work, we need to service our vehicles and fuel them properly. To the point, we need resources outside of ourselves for survival. Our health greatly depends on how well we manage *all* of these resources.

You may think of stock markets or political science when you hear about economics, but the word comes from the Greek *oikonomia*, meaning "household management," or the management of our personal resources. Each of us must be an economist of our energy expenditures, caloric intake, daily expenses, and material supplies. As we age, we often take on more responsibilities as spouses, parents, managers, coaches, bosses, and mentors—extending our decisions to include the welfare of family members and coworkers. Simple miscalculations can lead to discomfort. No one likes to find themselves with an empty toilet paper roll. But larger miscalculations land people in debt, bankruptcy, divorce, and consequences that are often avoidable if we approach our personal economics with the same honesty and curiosity as our spiritual practice.

Formal meditation practice offers a snapshot of what is replaying in our nervous systems. When everything else stops, you are better able to sense where your energy is going. We must ask ourselves if these thought patterns are worth the amount of energy they demand. We only have so much attention to give before we exhaust ourselves. At the fundamental level, this is economics: managing the amount of energy we are willing to forgo and measuring the reward we receive in return for that energy expenditure.

You can begin by identifying which patterns in your mental space drain too much energy. How many of them are true? There are likely a few thought balloons you can pop with ease by applying a little reason. Then you can begin to downsize the attention given to thoughts outside the present moment, particularly fears, judgments, and doubts. This cuts through the noise and frees up some space. Sometimes a little space is all we need for things to fall back into place. Hopefully, the space also gives us a new vantage point to refocus our energy on other issues.

The unyielding parts of our lives are where our pressures and stressors emerge from, typically surrounding our obligations. While it often seems that these responsibilities pose as large obstacles to our awakening, they are usually the challenges that lead us to greater spiritual depths.

One of those challenges usually revolves around money. Chögyam Trungpa Rinpoche referred to money as "green energy," which better depicts the nature of money as a potential for resources, instead of a metric of worth. Many of us are unskillful with green energy, few of us are truly taught how to work with it, and our inadequacies handling it leads us to demonize it. Money is necessary. It transfers energy through agreed value, creating safety for us to trade resources and coexist peacefully.

Before money or currency, we bartered. Each trade had its own value, but often deals were not on equal terms. For example, four pumpkins for one axe may be a good trade for a blacksmith who could make a new axe tomorrow but a terrible deal for a lumberjack who needs his axe for work each day. It is difficult to agree that one axe is worth four pumpkins, especially if that is all we had to trade. In economics, we call these differences in perceived value *opportunity costs*: the subjective, personal values that we assign resources in a given situation. The lumberjack has a much higher opportunity cost letting go of his axe than the blacksmith.

Here is another example of opportunity cost: If I offer you a sandwich when you are not hungry, it's unlikely that I could get you to buy it, even for a good price, let alone overpay for it. Your value of the sandwich is low because your stomach is full. But if I offered you the same sandwich when you had not eaten all day, it would likely be of interest, and if you were starving, you may even overpay to secure it for dinner. The sandwich itself has not changed, but our perceived value of it does, depending on our state of depletion when we come upon the offer. Before currency, it was easy to take advantage of those who had bad timing or few quality possessions to trade. We often forget that we used to pillage each other when opportunity costs equated poorly and trades went ugly.

Money creates a system of equality in which you can trade your labors and goods for a universal medium. Even though the value of things we trade will still be subjective, we can come to terms on equal grounds. Money can be saved, and it can carry you through ups and downs if managed properly. Currency also promotes cooperation, because we perceive the value of money as a group. Paper money has no value in itself. Put a bunch of it in a box and watch nothing happen. It offers some mental security to know it is there, but if you keep adding money to the box, at some point it will not create additional benefits. Money does not make us happy. It is useless, even destructive, if not properly utilized. Green energy must be spent wisely to obtain the supplies necessary to meet our challenges. Feeling comfortable and secure is what makes us happy, not the money itself. We need to save up for the big expenditures and keep some on the side for a rainy day. We cannot afford to be frivolous with our energy, especially when longer periods of discipline are necessary to achieve our goals.

When we accurately manage our resources, we keep ourselves nourished and maintain a sense of balance. You negotiate from a position of strength and can value resources and opportunities clearly, unclouded by any desperation. Our skills, discipline, and responsible behaviors will determine if our green energy is used efficiently or squandered. Life requires you to look at each expenditure with honesty. We often overspend unnecessarily. We waste, overpay for convenience, and continuously overvalue status and luxury possessions. We overlook expenditures of green energy and act like they have no karmic impact because we can make more money someday. No action goes without consequence. Every moment is an expenditure, a form of depletion. Practicing good economics is ensuring we receive appropriate value in return for those expenditures. Fortunes of all kinds are built one good decision at a time.

We may feel limited in this moment, but each day offers opportunities to finish with a little extra, reducing our deficit. It requires keeping a proper record of your actions and expenditures. We need to manage risks with their rewards, as we gamble today's resources to maintain stability tomorrow. Too often we choose short-term pleasures over handling our obligations properly. We must be mindful of wasting resources on forms of escapism that give little benefit in return. Living in the present moment does not mean being foolhardy about the future. You should not spend what you cannot afford, whether it is time, energy, or money. Living for today should include a certain amount of planning for tomorrow.

When you are practicing well, your correct actions will lend you spare energy accumulated through less conflict and resistance. This can be more physical energy, but it can also be additional money, skills, time, information, or trust. When we work with karma properly, we waste less, and the extra savings add up. Developing ourselves from within, we need less from the outside world to maintain our meditation, and resources last longer and stretch further. Retrieving the maximum value out of our possessions is a great way to practice sustainability and gratitude. After that, we must accept how everything has its limits.

Even if you are ultra-wealthy, you are still mortal, susceptible to accidents, illnesses, and plenty of variables that money cannot save us from. Life is limited. We only have so much room in our stomachs for food, so much energy in a day, and so much time on Earth. We must work consciously within the edges of our limitations regardless of our ambitions or means. These confines are not always obstacles we must overcome. You must play within the rules of the game. Having limits helps us know when we have had enough and helps us refrain from wasting resources. We are still healthy competitors pushing each other to achieve greatness, but we recognize that for every great success, sacrifices were made to achieve it, balancing the scales.

What assets are realistically at your disposal? Do you have the awareness to harness them? When we are open to the world of possibilities, we are rich in every moment, regardless of our limitations. There is abundance all around us. We often have more options than we notice, especially when moving too fast or fixating too far in the distance. We may fail to perceive options and falsely conclude they do not exist. Abundance is not about wealth but the full awareness to recognize, create, and capitalize on opportunities.

Practicing personal economics is an everyday affair. Even when you are well stocked, food spoils, wood turns to ash, the seasons change, and there is need to replenish. While we cannot predict the future, we can reasonably prepare for whatever comes next. We should be comfortable with what resources are available and know how to use them. Being responsible does not mean that you have every supply imaginable or a plan for every situation. Stability comes from practicing good personal economics, working well with green energy, skillfully with karma, and a mentality of abundance and resourcefulness. If we have properly met our responsibilities and use our energy wisely, we should be on a good footing for whatever life throws our way. There is no version of stability where you do not have to put in the work. It remains good practice to hope for the best but prepare for the worst.

It is a common misconception that choosing peace means never going to war. We may not choose if war comes. We must be ready to thwart those who wish ill upon us. We must be strong enough to protect what is precious. The warrior spirit does not seek aggression but harnesses power to refute threatening advances on the innocent. More often than violent threats of war, social and economic responsibilities usually reflect our battlefields, but our primal priorities remain the same: be aware, have a plan, and be prepared to drop the plan and adapt to whatever opens up in front of us.

In every moment energy swirls around you like arrows zipping about. These figurative pointed whirls include everything from desires, ambitions, and emotions to unforeseeable circumstances, accidents, and even the weather. With arrows flying in all directions, we are bound to get caught in the crossfire of a world filled with intentions, no matter how much awareness we embody.

Sometimes we are struck by unfortunate events just for being in the wrong place at the wrong time. You can shake them off and not take it personally. Other times we may have avoided arrows not meant for us but met a jarring surprise because we were not paying attention. In the worst of it, shots are aimed at us deliberately, painfully, and destructively. But whenever an arrow hits you, there is a choice whether or not to raise your bow and fire back.

The awakened person does not return the shot. We are not martyrs nor should we allow others to wound us intentionally, but our response should reduce additional harm or negative karmic momentum. We cannot always avoid conflict or challenges, but we are always responsible for how we handle our bow, even when arrows strike us in uncomfortable places. You must develop the thick skin and the warrior spirit to stay vigilant and walk through the fray. By slowing down and proceeding with correct action, we can encounter fewer arrows. Our meditation serves as our first line of defense. Discernment is our shield, evading what does not serve us, never actively seeking battle. Each motion is calculated and deliberate, void of unnecessary risks. We leave enough space to take our time, avoiding foolish mistakes that can be prevented by acting with preparedness and mindfulness.

You cannot hide from struggle and pray no arrows strike you. That is not an awakened life. Each of the practices we discussed recharge us to get back out there. Awakening requires us to treat each arrow as an opportunity for correct action and openness. If we find ourselves repeatedly dealing with arrows, we likely need to review. You may have little room to maneuver, making you an easy target. An overcrowded lifestyle can leave us feeling boxed in, and we are not in our right minds when we feel trapped. Sometimes we need space to duck out of the way. Other times we need space to ensure that our actions align with our intentions, to withdraw our arrow, even when we raise our bow automatically.

Meditation practice affords us inner space to explore, wander, and be available for alternatives. How many times have we acted the same way while expecting a different result? How many arrows have we fired that made the situation worse? Our reaction can be more terrible than the offense itself. Remove arrows with dignity and nurse wounds before they get worse. Procrastination only leads to additional pain and suffering.

Seeing things clearly through your meditation practice reduces the likelihood of reacting poorly to challenges in relationships, taking things personally, or becoming overwhelmed by circumstances outside of your control. We handle our obligations and refrain from firing more arrows into an unpredictable world. We ensure that we have the necessary resources to meet our responsibilities. Only once our obligations are met do we factor in our pleasures.

We are warriors, economists, dynamos. The future is ours to harvest together. We each have to take responsibility for dreaming the world into being, to do our part in peacefully creating paradise on Earth.

REFLECTIONS

Am I honoring all of my responsibilities?

What are the areas of my life that are inflexible?

How can I better support my efforts in inflexible areas?

Where can I do less? Where must I do more?

Are there two versions of me?

RESPONSIBILITY

What are the things that make me raise my bow without thinking?

Can I gain more flexibility in my schedule? Or do I need to be more flexible to make things work?

Do I meet the unexpected and challenging parts of life with openness?

*in uncertainty, practice patience
in loss, practice gratitude
in fear, practice presence
all challenges come to pass,
just keep practicing.*

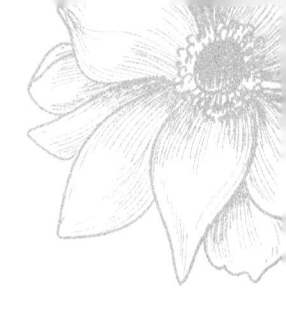

9

ACCEPTANCE

THERE IS A POINT when we must stop seeking wisdom teachings and really focus on living our practice. By now, I hope that you are starting to see the pattern of awakening as a series of conscious acts, steadily shaping us into peaceful beings, living harmoniously with the world around us. The path is gradual, punctuated when teachings and experiences mix together, illustrating life beyond words.

Each of us who commits long enough to spiritual practice goes through a dry spell of growth, where we feel like we have plateaued. Wisdom progresses more like rolling hills than climbing straight to a prolific peak of realization. We learn as much in the valley as we do at the summit. Even when we have illuminating moments, they are a culmination of us doing the work. The work is not some exotic technique that snaps us out of our current reality to the "truth." There is no magic. Awakening is skillfully managing your emotions and interactions exactly where you are and accepting things exactly as they are, in the present moment. Let us reemphasize that the awareness we are cultivating is available with any formal meditation practice technique. The priority is to commit to the redundancy of the practice and bear witness to the subtle changes.

If you shed one flake at a time, it takes a while before the progress is obvious. Then suddenly, deeper questions bubble up to the surface. *How does a seed become a flower? How foolish is the wave that sees itself apart from the ocean?* Each of the practices we have explored help us stay present to the experience, all the way through the results. When we succeed, we try to repeat those skillful actions, and when we fail, we learn the lessons and make the necessary adjustments to better work with karma. This task is harder than usual for us facing the unprecedented distractions of the computer era.

A key difference between our lives today and previous societies is our ability to witness each other. Unlike our ancestors, we have new connections through technology, allowing us to spend a lot of time digitally with people with whom we may never have any personal relationship. Without a real two-way relationship in which we also exert influence (think mirror neurons), these one-way forms of communication leave us as consumers. Too much media does not seem to serve us well, whether or not we agree with the opinions we are observing. The Internet changed the way we communicate, and honest and primal, many of its first uses were to cry out for help.

ACCEPTANCE

Social media has become a place to display terrible injustices, and these are often the stories that flood the headlines. This has led to side effects that were impossible to foresee, from the mass exposure to suffering beyond our personal experience and its impact on our empathic brains. We now learn of the tribulations of cultures across the globe, most of which exert little to no influence on our lives directly. The collective misery can seem insurmountable. This is a new phenomenon: the sense of helplessness from witnessing the suffering of those whom we will never touch. It is happening on an international level.

Each society has its own obstacles and challenges it must face in order to grow. It is the natural way. Instead of wallowing in the negative state of things, we must accept things as they are and return to the present moment in front of us, where we can participate directly. Acceptance does not guarantee that we are comfortable with the situation, but knowledge of a problem does not necessarily make it our fight, particularly the ones that do not directly affect us. This is not to be defeatist or dismissive of issues that matter, but we would be wiser and more effective to concentrate our efforts on the things we can actually impact. Those situations are likely to be much closer to home, offline, and where your attention is needed most.

Each of us must learn from our direct experience. You can likely remember a situation in which you had been warned or were told to stay away but proceeded anyhow, and only after it turned into a blunder. . . then you got the message. We often need to learn in our own way. It may be tempting to try to shield those we care about from facing misfortunes, insisting we are helping them avoid harm. But you have no right to take another's pain away. You may be denying them a crucial lesson. Do not tolerate harm befalling someone but practice protection in ways that allow lessons to still reach their intended recipients. We can be available to help others, but we should be mindful of inserting our aid in places where it is not asked of us. Accept that you are only responsible for your participation, not the outcome.

Life is not typically as complicated as we make it out to be. But there are times when we are unskillful in the first round, and instead of admitting the mistake and changing course, we compound the problem. We may feel ourselves backpedaling, getting defensive, and hiding behind the notion that "it's complicated." Too often, it is *not* complicated we are simply afraid to admit that we do not know the answer. No one has all the answers. We each have to deal with the suspicion that we may never fully understand life, regardless of our belief systems.

Seeking an understanding of the great mysteries is part of the human experience. We seek proof of our beliefs in order to create a stable sense of how to live. We create ethics of conformity so we can accurately anticipate each other. We want things to be reliable so we can form trust, attempting to create certainty in an uncertain world. This stability needs ongoing cooperation, maintenance, and adaptation. When you are lucky enough to reach a space of steadiness and comfort, enjoy it, but do not overextend yourself to maintain it. A lot of unnecessary despair befalls those trying to make things permanent in an ever-changing world. Nothing lasts forever, the good times or the bad. Our unwillingness to let go and accept impermanence only deepens our resistance and thus our suffering.

Leaving space for the unpredictable is crucial to keeping our ego in check. When plans are foiled, ego screams. When plans are flexible, you can adjust without suffering. Sometimes this flexibility is referred to as surrendering. It may be hard to digest if we associate surrender with giving up, quitting, or failure. But we are not forgoing our autonomy, only surrendering to the outcome. It is not something that we can possess anyway, only something we can get attached to inappropriately. No more can be asked of us than trying our best, and if we can look in the mirror and know we gave it our greatest effort, all that is left is acceptance when providence does not come our way. The universe does not owe us an explanation.

Our practice should be a source of strength during moments of uncertainty. Most of our worries never come to pass. Remembering negativity bias, our minds may exaggerate problems to ready us for disaster. But what is the likelihood of the situation we are preparing for? We must be wary of cluttering our minds with paranoid worries that have a minuscule probability of becoming reality.

There are times when you make fastidious plans, execute well, and the outcome is still not in your favor. There are forces greater than ourselves and we are not in complete control (traffic jams!). Awakening requires us to accept the inexplicable and make peace with it. Gratitude is crucial to maintaining openness when situations develop in ways we do not understand. If we can appreciate the moments when life conspires for our benefit, we are less likely to wail when our intentions get stymied. Leave space for accidents to happen. Leave space for things to grow in unexpected ways.

By slowing down and savoring each moment, we can live 10,000 lifetimes in one body and meet our final moments with grace. Death seeks us all. None of us escape it. Allow the unfolding mystery to be exciting! Who knows what blessings are still to come?

REFLECTIONS

What in my life do I have trouble accepting?

Do I acknowledge and respect the forces greater than myself?

Do I accept that all things are not explainable?

Do I truly need the answer to be happy?

Do I swim against the tide or do I go with the flow? How is it going?

Am I surrendering?

Am I being of service to others or do I usually take?

How do trees practice acceptance?

not escape,
LIBERATE!

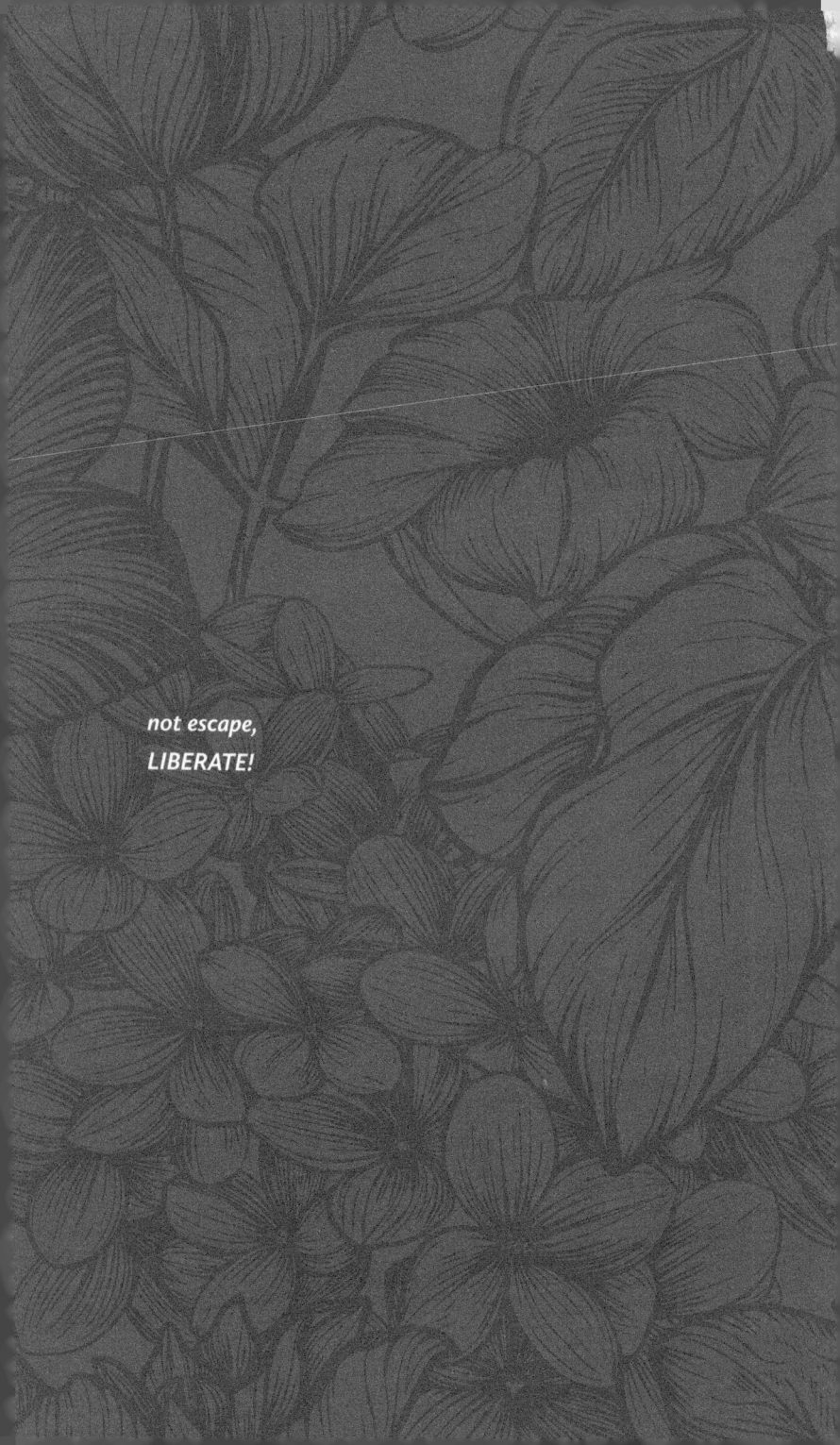

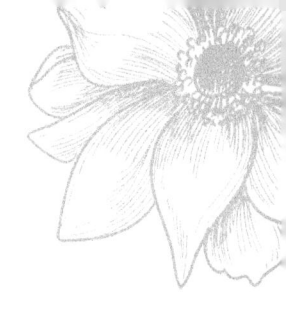

10

GENEROSITY

AS WE APPROACH OUR final key, let us take a moment to summarize how the keys and practices we have discussed interweave and build upon each other. You start (or restart) by getting honest, admitting your flaws, accepting what you cannot change, and motivating yourself to cleanse your *stuff*. You experience life as it is, instead of living with expectations. You review your daily choices and their impacts. Local, seasonal, organic foods provide dense nutrients to keep your energy high and health balanced, with the least stress on natural resources. Adequate rest and time in the delta wave state of deep sleep maximizes 3R Mode of repairing, refreshing, and recording. Exercising daily with an appropriate amount of fitness keeps your body running efficiently and helps it ease into restorative sleep. Your habits give a direct line into karma through daily repetition, showing whether you are positively or negatively altering your well-being. You remember the gap between noticing and fixing and continuously make refinements in sustainable ways that lead to lasting transformation.

Meditation practice is an opportunity to stop everything and reset. You bring your attention to thoughts and perceptions, nonjudgmentally noticing what keeps replaying in your consciousness. Staying curious and learning new things, you practice cultivating joy. Maintaining supportive habits focused on the positive aspects of your situation keeps you open-minded. You maintain flexibility, physically and emotionally, by counterbalancing negativity bias and keeping your nervous system from getting overstimulated. You accept your part in a larger system and stay in harmony with all beings, including the plants and animals. You cultivate positive, non-harming relationships by honoring your responsibilities. When you do your part, it is easier to accept what you cannot change.

How well we maximize opportunities will determine if we have the space to make our own choices—to decide between options, assess a situation on our own terms, make vital changes to stop habitual patterns, and re-ground ourselves when necessary. Inner freedom is earned through balance, diligence, and resourcefulness. If we do not spread ourselves too thin or live above our means, we should have abundant energy to share with others. We share our abundance by acting with compassion, being of service, and practicing generosity.

As you commit to your practice, it may be tempting to ask, how do I know that I am doing any of this correctly? How can I be sure I am in meditation if I do not feel relaxed or peaceful? If you start looking around and comparing your journey to others in search of a baseline, you are headed for trouble. You need to start exactly where you are, which is only relevant to you.

Here is a secret that social media rarely shares: many of us first embark on the spiritual path because we are suffering. Our situation forces us to concede that we are off-balance and our poor choices are unsustainable. We cannot compare ourselves to those at different points of their spiritual journeys. We must find our own way. Journals are great for chronicling our transformation. If you make a little progress each day, it may not be noticeable how far you have come until you cringe at an old entry.

So much of our suffering is not real; it only comes from feeling like we never have enough, whether it is not enough time or not enough *stuff* to fill up our time. Scarcity triggers feeling threatened, invoking the fight-or-flight response, survivalism, and tribalism. These primal urges can be very destructive, leading to the selfishness, competitiveness, and combativeness we often witness in the world. In order to calm the fear that we never have enough, we must be more resourceful. This is the same panic that comes from swimming against the tide of karma. It is an acquired skill to change this perspective, to realize that you have everything you need right now to meet your challenges with ease and grace. It is not an absence of anything that causes pain, it is our presence of mind. Even if we are really short on time or resources at this moment, it is unlikely causing us as much suffering as the resistance created by wasting energy desiring alternative circumstances.

Remember: **Suffering = Pain x Resistance**. Craving, attachment, desire for alternatives, and escapism are all forms of the same illness: hiding (resistance) from the present and not accepting it for exactly what it is in this moment. Pain may happen without our consent, but resistance is within our control. Not all moments feel good, and that is okay. Nothing in life—including awakening—is all tulips and roses. It is a common pitfall to be overprotective or antisocial when beginning to witness the suffering around us, whether on our streets or in the news. The blinders are taken off, our empathy increases, and we notice how much work there is still to be done. It can feel like pain is everywhere, suffering all around. Even if that were true, we cannot take on the world all at once. The removal of the veil does not lead to the unsheathing of the sword.

A call to action in the face of such adversity can leave us feeling isolated. Allow nature to fill in the gaps, becoming a companion and source of stability. There is no greater teacher of the bigger picture, interconnectedness, and impermanence. We are never truly alone. We must remain with one foot in the shared reality, no matter the discomfort. If we find ourselves overwhelmed and hiding in cocoons because the outside world is unsupportive of our practice, we will not emerge as butterflies to clearer skies. Instead, our resistance will fester, and we will rot.

Awakening is the journey of learning to consciously act in meditation, regardless of the conditions. Anyone can treat daily tasks as an opportunity to practice operating in meditation in each action. When you let go of seeking gurus or exotic mystical states and focus on your *stuff* and the immediate world in front of you, there is plenty of material for practice, right here and now.

When we practice good personal economics, there is a tipping point where we begin to operate from a place of extra energy and abundance. We are well balanced in ourselves, wise with our energy to meet our needs, and this should create extra energy and opportunities to share with others, whether it is time, attention, money, resources, or knowledge. There are infinite ways that we can share with each other. When you have a solid understanding of your personal needs, it is much easier to assess what you can give without personal interruption. This may seem very transactional, but the survival parts of our brain will not deprive us of necessities without good reason.

Awakening does not ask you to offer what you do not have to give. If someone asks something that you cannot provide, say no. Being of service is like lifting someone over our heads. If the request depletes us in ways we cannot replenish, or we are on a bad footing when service is asked of us, we may become weak and collapse during the lift, potentially hurting ourselves and those who sought the help. If we want to raise others up, we must have a strong, well-grounded foundation. We need to be honest about what we can contribute and not make promises we cannot uphold. It is a terrible curse to try to reclaim energies we should not have parted with, especially if pride or embarrassment leave us suffering in secret. There are ways you can help where you do not need to question the lines between being selfless and foolish.

Instead of feeling blameworthy or inadequate when we are not well positioned to meet a request, focus on what services *can* be offered. Another option may be exactly what the situation needs. Guilt should only arise when we are wasteful, selfish, have the ability to share but refuse, or close down. It is not the same as being protective or wise about your energy. You know the difference between being lazy about participating and when you truly cannot (or should not) meet a request.

We are not required to suffer for the benefit of others. If your energy is not freely given, it is taken. There is resistance. It increases suffering. Usually when something is taken from us, it is followed by an expectation of reimbursement, leaving us waiting for repayment from the person, situation, or some sort of kickback from the universe—none of which is guaranteed. When we give what we are comfortable contributing, we do not look for anything in return. When you give with caveats or conditions, it opens the door for disappointment or worse. Our practices help us maintain balance and poise so we can respond when called upon—and we will be called. It is inevitable that we will always need to help and share with each other, and it is less likely that a task will ask too much of us if we are operating from a state of meditation.

Generosity is willingly giving our energy to others without looking for retribution or repayment. A poignant form of generosity is compassion: the reduction of suffering by sharing or removing pain and resistance. It is often misunderstood to be feeling sympathetic and sorrowful for a person or situation, but it is an action, going directly to the point of friction and energetically diffusing the suffering. Our meditation practice is a form of self-compassion. You take time out to notice exactly where there is pain or resistance and try to let it go. When caught in a thought loop, you have to take conscious action to stop feeding it energy. Feeling sorry for yourself is not the same as empowering yourself by practicing acceptance. In the same way, compassion is active.

When we console a friend who is furious, they vent and we can take on some of their fury. It is not our anger, so we do not claim it, but help diffuse it so it does not further poison our friend. Perhaps you bring joy and support to your friend until the fury burns itself out. Whether we view the energy exchange as taking or giving, we help our friend reduce their pain or resistance by offering our understanding. This exchange will deplete us, but we do so willingly, without resistance, so we do not suffer for it.

You may be incapable of removing the pain, yet we can fortify each other, often through the simple act of listening. But if we are only a blank wall to scream at without offering genuine support, the fury bounces off without diminishing and likely leads to our friend yelling at someone else, spreading the fury until its energy is properly diffused. But compassion actively reduces the potential for further harm by scattering negative karmic momentum.

Generosity is a selfless spreading of joy, giving without any attachment, like a person entering a room and throwing candy to children. There is no self in what we give away, because it is not ours to begin with, we are only agents of prosperity. We are blessed in so many ways that we may forget how incredible life is at its core. The inherent quality of life is abundance.

The warrior spirit remains strong and generous by harnessing the power of the universe without depleting internal energy. When we learn how to dance in the wind, we do not fear walking headfirst into the tempest. It may be another opportunity, one that may not have been obvious or available to us before, but the awakened mind sees more, feels more, and connects more.

When we practice generosity, we share our deeper vision with the world, and we lead with love. You reduce resistance just by your presence, your joy. You radiate. Radiance is what attracts people to us, to our spirit, and to the steadiness of the awakened state. We embody meditation in all of our actions, sharing our wisdom by living the path authentically.

REFLECTIONS

Which of the ten keys provide stability for me?

Where do I need to focus my energy?

Who is someone in my life that exemplifies generosity?

Where am I still resisting?

How often do I feel in abundance?

Can I be more open to possibilities?

Am I generous?

Do I lead with love?

You have everything you need right now to awaken.

The awakened one maintains meditation in their actions, regardless of the conditions, a state of being that we are most likely to inhabit by honoring and maintaining these ten keys.

Be here now, and just keep practicing.
I wish you all the best on your spiritual journey.
Good luck!

THANK YOU

IT TOOK ME TEN years from the first words jotted down until the book you hold was complete. Thank you for taking the time to read it and for giving me purpose. I would like to acknowledge a short but important list of people, without whom it would never have manifested.

Thank you, all my teachers, living and deceased, who illuminated the path for me to follow, specifically my yoga teachers Raji Thron, Fran Ubertini, Carol Bowman, and Kelly Solloway, and additionally Elena Brower, Rodney Yee, and Dharma Mittra. Thank you Chögyam Trungpa Rinpoche, Thich Nhat Hahn, Ram Dass, Rick Hanson, and Stephen Batchelor, for even though we have never met, you illuminated these teachings through your writings in ways that changed my life forever. Your advice continues to challenge me daily, and I am eternally grateful.

Thank you, Mom and Dad, for providing the foundation for my ethics, and thank you to my sister, Jackie, and family members who put up with me through the dark times. I know that we live in an era where too few have the stability of a strong family structure, and I know how much work it takes to be a supportive family. A surprising amount of this text are things I first learned at the dinner table.

Thank you to all my students and friends in the yoga community, for participating in my journey and allowing me to experiment on you. I think this book is the worthy accumulation of our trials, even if it seems rather far away from the early years of doing yoga under the influence of essential oils, colored lights, and drums. A special thank you to my friend Nisar, for always believing in me and first insisting that I should condense the madness into something useful.

Thank you, Jennifer Kasius, for editing said madness into a language digestible to others and for challenging me when it got too far out. Your kindness is echoed in many ways within this text.

Thank you, to the book formatting team at Becky's Graphic Design®, I am so grateful for the ways you have enhanced this project and made it beautiful.

And lastly, but certainly not least, thank you to my wife, Casey. Without your patience and insistence, this book would likely not exist. It is your strength and fortitude that this work really reflects, as you propped up your husband, an emotional roller coaster of a human being, and ensured that I finished what I started. Should this book have the impact you believe it will, the victory will be yours. I look forward to continuing to practice together now as parents, as the next chapter of spiritual evolution begins.

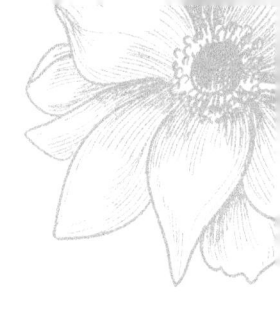

A GUIDE TO EXTENDED SPIRITUAL PRACTICE AT HOME:

HOMEGROWN RETREATS

I HOPE THAT THE ten keys have resonated with you: that you've been able to identify areas of support in your life, and that you have some newfound awareness. But what I also hope (in a fun, non-malicious way!) is that something rubbed you the wrong way. There are a lot of (subtle?) challenges throughout the book, and taking time out to acknowledge what those things are is important. There are many teachings that I hated the first time I heard them because they made me aware of my inadequate efforts. They became new catchphrases for the annoying voices in my head. But I did not let the discomfort turn me away from the challenges. It can be difficult to see things clearly when we are just trying to survive. One of the most effective ways I have found to hit the reset button is to take some time for a personal retreat.

Retreating is taking time to practice awakening, by setting aside distraction-free time to practice meditation in all our actions. From extended meditation engagement, we have opportunities to experience the natural healing qualities of the body and return to balance. It is a highly customizable healing art form, and this is a simple guide to get you off the ground. As someone who personally loves to retreat and has spent a lot of weekends teaching in forests and at festivals far away from everyday life, I can attest to the refreshing power of consciously breaking away from our routines to reset. And as someone also running a small business, I know the challenges and disappointments of returning to an urban grind of rude, mindless people after feeling so clear and ready for a brighter world to emerge.

Too many of us come right to the edge, or crash and burn, before we acknowledge that we need a break. We cannot constantly fight to get back into balance. Retreating can create the space necessary for healing our inner and outer worlds, to plug back into natural energies and fully recharge.

It may be an ongoing challenge to have opportunities to practice, especially after the pandemic disrupted so many of our communities. As we went into our cocoons, some of us thrived in the solitude, but many of us did not. We were cut off from our mentors, teachers, friends, and communities, and we lost support systems that we counted on. Finding ourselves on our own, many of us have the fortitude to do the work but may not have a clear path for what to do next. In these instances, I think the practice should return to the basics of focusing on health and energy levels highlighted in the ten keys. It seems that we are always most vulnerable when our energy is out of balance. A personal retreat is a great way to return to balance, particularly if we focus on practicing meditation.

APPENDIX I

FIVE BASICS OF AN EFFECTIVE HOME RETREAT

A WELL-DESIGNED RETREAT SHOULD leave you feeling fresh and rejuvenated from the experience, typically focusing and exploring a singular theme. Regardless of the topic or the length of your practice, each retreat should reflect these five basics to ensure you are filling your cup:

1. **Break from Routine**

    When we go into retreat, we are intentionally breaking away from our habitual behaviors, whether it's for a few hours or a few months. Find a place where you can be quiet and undisturbed for the entire duration of your experience. When we retreat to a new destination, the breakaway is easier, but when we are home, it may not be as simple to distance ourselves from our family, friends, and social responsibilities. Make arrangements with loved ones so that you can shut off your devices and disconnect without guilt or fear. If our body is in one place but our mind is in another, we are not really retreating or in meditation.

    Find a practice area that brings a sense of peace and relaxation naturally. We need to be in the present moment to gain this headspace, and that includes feeling safe and comfortable in our practice area. Retreats encourage us to slow down, to be removed from our responsibilities, to get distance from our emotional triggers, and to simply relax. Don't overstuff the schedule; leave space to rest and go slowly. Leave plenty of room for slow transitions. Enjoy the outdoors. Practice silence. Listen.

We want to stay in our state of meditation as much as possible during retreat, so choose your location wisely. Think ahead about bathroom breaks. Plan for other potential distractions and how to avoid them. Whenever planning a personal retreat, you should make it your top priority to find a supportive space with minimal distractions. It may require traveling, or you may need familiar terrain to find tranquility. That is completely your choice. The key is breaking far enough away from our routines to feel it, to be able to lean into our retreat for the full duration of the experience, stay present to any internal shifts, complete our practices, and heal.

2. **Study & Reflection Materials**

Typically, on a guided retreat, a master teacher gives lessons and guidance throughout the experience to reinforce central themes and instruct practices. Substitute these instructions with your own chosen study materials, such as pre-recorded retreats, dharma talks, guided meditations, or lectures. Read sutras, poetry, and books. If you want someone to read to you, audiobooks can be paused, slowly digested, and enjoyed over the whole weekend. Fortunately for us in the age of technology, many retreats by master teachers have been recorded and can be purchased (and they are already broken down into lectures and practices).

Pick study materials in advance. If you plan to have a lot of formal practice, choose study material that is less time-consuming and more contemplative. If practicing less and relaxing more, you can enjoy the wisdom of a master teacher to serve as a central theme for your weekend.

Do not rush through your materials. Digest teachings slowly and reflect on what you are learning. Set specific times, give your full attention, and then pause and take a break, leaving room to absorb and explore. Studying should serve to complement the other parts of the retreat and should not be so ambitious that it feels like homework. It's okay to finish the materials after your retreat experience ends, in fact, it can be a great way to keep the momentum of the practice moving back into ordinary experience. Within the provided sample schedule, these will be your materials for the Study & Reflection section.

3. **Extended Formal Practice**

Typically, the biggest deviation from our normal routine during a retreat is the amount of formal practice each day. Depending on the experience we are creating, formal practice can include sitting meditation, movement practices like walking meditation, yoga asana, or chi gong, and self-care practices such as sound baths and abhyanga massage. What types of practice—and how much of it—will be the choice of each practitioner and will vary depending on our healing needs as we plan each experience. I've provided a sample schedule at the end of this section, where you'll find options for suggested formal practices, varying between sitting practice and additional movement options.

Plan out a challenging yet realistic schedule, and stick to it. Include movement throughout the day—especially if you are doing a lot of sitting practice—to keep yourself feeling fresh. Even if you want to focus on sitting practice, take breaks for your circulation and rotate between sitting and some sort of restorative movement in between sessions, preferably gentle yoga or walking meditation. Reserve mornings for rigorous movement practices to prepare the body for long periods of meditation and relaxed/restorative sequences to work out any stiffness in the evenings. Maintain silence as much as possible in between practices.

It's an extra step, but I highly recommend utilizing free smartphone apps such as Insight Timer to help sequence timers in advance. Set bells to sound at scheduled times, such as after 30 minutes for meditation, then another bell after a 10-minute movement break, and then another bell at the end of the next 30-minute sitting practice, and so on. Setting multiple bell timers can make for hitting the button once and allowing all retreaters to stay in meditation as the timers go off automatically, with no energy spent on anyone keeping time or resetting between sessions. Insight Timer even has different bells to signal different happenings during your experience. When my wife and I have our home retreat experiences, our bells are scheduled in blocks of 3-4 hours, so we can stay on schedule without having to look at a clock.

Remember that retreating is a healing act. Sometimes we need to break through, and sitting through the discomfort during meditation may be a necessary part of our process. But if it becomes too painful, then we are tormenting ourselves for no reason. If your body is not up for the challenge, your mind will be distracted, and little healing will come of it. Do not be embarrassed if you need to sit in a chair later in the day to give your hips or knees a break. Modify to meet your body's needs whenever necessary, and remember to keep focusing on maintaining a state of meditation.

Change the postures, make the modifications, but complete the practices and the schedule you set out in the beginning.

4. Mindful Eating

Guided retreats often include food as part of their experience to ensure that their guests are supported nutritionally. Extended practice includes resetting internally through our food choices, which play a large role in engaging the natural healing qualities of the body. Keep meals light and all-natural in between formal practices. Eating heavily, whether by eating too much or from heavy ingredients like meat and dairy, usually induces sleepiness. It may be an opportune time to try vegetarian cuisine and see if you feel any difference. Be mindful of your intake of caffeine, sugar, and other stimulating foods throughout the retreat (less is better). If you make a poor choice, let it serve as an opportunity to witness how that food makes you feel during practice and make a better choice next time.

Cooking and eating offer additional opportunities to practice maintaining our meditation while performing simple actions. At your home retreat (and in general), take control of your food whenever possible. Plan the menu, and gather all cooking utensils and ingredients in advance. Whether you are heading deep into the wilderness for a camping retreat or just hiding out in your bedroom, make it easy to prepare meals while sustaining meditation. Prepare food in silence and clean up completely after each meal. Too many of us do the eating but do not participate in the full process of cooking and cleaning up that is necessary to properly nourish ourselves. Leave no trace.

There have been retreats where I wanted to detox myself so I adhered to strict vegan menus and other times when we would cap off each night by *mindfully* chowing down luxurious desserts. The moment will call for what's right, and finding the balance of practice and pleasure will vary from each individual and retreat experience. But retreating should *not* be vacationing, even if there are long doses of relaxation. Vacationing can be an invitation to fulfill a set of desires and be indulgent. That's fine, and it can be very therapeutic, but it is not practice. Retreating is an active gesture of love, where we practice getting ourselves balanced and give ourselves the personal attention to make us better upon our return to the real world. A retreat is training, practicing being in a state of meditation in all of our actions. Retreating is an act of healing, and pleasure can be important to healing, as long as we make good decisions.

5. **Relaxation & Self-Care Rituals**

Your retreat schedule should be invigorating without being exhausting. If a weekend of seemingly endless practice seems intimidating, try balancing practice with self-care rituals and quiet relaxation. Often less is more, and simply removing ourselves from stimulating environments helps relax us naturally. Leave extra space for transitions and maintain a relaxed pace. It can take a while to unwind if we are coming from a place of intensity before retreating. We also do not want to jump back into the mix without proper time to transition.

Often when we take time to reset ourselves, the reality of our pre-retreat imbalances becomes glaringly clear. That is part of the process, to notice the imbalances. But simply noticing something does not mean it can immediately be undone. Be kind to yourself. Remember that you are bringing a refreshed sense of awareness to the situation. Bring clear energy to those areas and use your newfound peace to support your wellness and make adjustments.

When you need a break, slow down, sit quietly, and reflect. Stretch out or prep your next meal extra slowly. Get a massage, or if that's out of reach, learn about the tradition of self-massage called abhyanga. Try listening to a sound bath, journaling, diffusing essential oils, or just lying outside and staring at the sky. Only participate in activities that maintain or enhance your state of meditation. Stay silent and allow the quiet to come over you.

Nature is your best companion on retreat. Tea and cozy blankets are also highly recommended.

Refrain from activities that will break your concentration such as phone calls, checking messages, unplanned snacking, or listening to loud music. Bring only the things you need for your retreat and nothing else to distract you. Let the senses shut off, give yourself little to do, and simply be present to the world around you. Breaking away includes all of our habitual, auto-pilot reactions to our possessions and environment. It is an essential part of the retreating process, stepping far enough away from our daily habits so that we can see them more clearly. Sometimes the clearest way to see this is to indulge in doing nothing for a while.

Keeping these five basics in mind, we maintain our state of being, health, and environment, setting us up for a successful recharge during our retreat experience. Now let's take a look at what we will need and plan out a schedule.

RECOMMENDED GEAR LIST

<u>Minimum:</u>

- ☐ A quiet space to practice
- ☐ Yoga mat or blanket to establish your practice area
- ☐ Cushion, zafu, zabuton, bench, or chair for seated meditation
- ☐ Adjustable timer or digital alarm/timer
- ☐ A meditation technique you are comfortable practicing
- ☐ Extra drinking water
- ☐ Study materials
- ☐ Comfortable, loose clothing for practices
- ☐ Downloads/paper copies for movement sequences

<u>For longer retreats also include:</u>

- ☐ Food ingredients
- ☐ Cooking utensils
- ☐ Sleepwear and toiletries
- ☐ Light, all-natural snacks

Optional:

- ☐ Yoga props such as blocks or bolsters for restorative practices
- ☐ Additional blankets for outdoor practice and lounging
- ☐ Proper shoes for walking meditation in your chosen terrain
- ☐ Sound Bath recordings, poetry readings, or additional lectures
- ☐ Tea or herbal tisanes
- ☐ Incense, essential oils, abhyanga oils
- ☐ Journals, writing materials
- ☐ Headphones / speakers

SAMPLE WEEKEND RETREAT SCHEDULE

THIS IS ONE IDEA for a retreat, a weekend template for working people, but it is entirely up to you how you would like to plan your experience. All the times are adjustable to meet your needs and ambitions. For retreats only a few hours or half-day, try the Friday or Sunday schedules. For single full-day retreats, try the Saturday schedule. For weekend retreats, use the suggested schedule in full, and for extended retreats, repeat the Saturday schedule each day, until ending with the Sunday schedule on the final day.

FRIDAY NIGHT

- ☐ Prepare practice area.
- ☐ Ensure you have all cooking ingredients, supplies, and gear.
- ☐ Sign off with outside world.
- ☐ Prepare your sacred space.
- ☐ Set up your remaining gear for easy transitions.
- ☐ Officially begin retreat with a bow.

1. **After dinner:**
   Gentle Movement *(10—30 minutes)* and Sitting Meditation *(30—60 minutes)*.

2. **Choose:**
   Study and Reflection *(30—90 minutes)*

   <u>or</u>

   Walking Meditation/Gentle Yoga *(10—15 minutes)* and Sitting Meditation *(30—60 minutes)* and Walking/Yoga *(10—15 minutes)*.

3. **Close practice with:**
   Sitting Meditation *(30—60 minutes)* and head to bed.

SATURDAY

1. **Wake Up Early:**
   Sitting Meditation *(30—45 minutes)*.

2. **Choose:**
   Morning Yoga, raise the heart rate! *(60—90 minutes)*

   <u>or</u>

   Walking Meditation/Gentle Yoga *(10—15 minutes)* and Sitting Meditation *(30—60 minutes)* and Walking/Yoga *(10—15 minutes)*.

3. **Close practice with:**
   Sitting Meditation *(30—60 minutes)*.

4. **Breakfast** *(preferably in silence)*.

5. **Then:**
   Study and Reflection *(60—90 minutes)* and Seated Meditation *(30—60 minutes)*.

6. **Lunch then:**
   Walking Meditation (*in nature if possible*).

7. **Then:**
   Study and Reflection (*60—90 minutes*) and Seated Meditation (*30—60 minutes*).

8. **Choose:**
   Evening Yoga, Restorative or Yin (*60—90 minutes*)

   or

   Sitting Meditation (*30—60 minutes*) and Walking Meditation/Gentle Yoga (*15 minutes*) and Sitting Meditation (*30—60 minutes*) and Walking/Yoga (*15 minutes*).

9. **Closing:**
   Sitting Meditation (*30—60 minutes*).

10. **After Dinner:**
    Self-Care Rituals (*30—60 minutes*).

11. **Closing:**
    Sitting Meditation or Sound Bath (*30—60 minutes*) and head to bed.

SUNDAY

1. **Wake Up Early:**
   Sitting Meditation (*30—45 minutes*).

2. **Choose:**
   Morning Yoga, relax and rejuvenate (*60—90 minutes*)

   or

   Walking Meditation/Gentle Yoga (*15 minutes*) and Sitting Meditation (*30—60 minutes*) and Walking/Yoga (*15 minutes*).

3. **Closing:**
   Sitting Meditation (*30—60 minutes*).

4. **Breakfast then:**
   Study and Reflection (*60—90 minutes*) and Seated Meditation (*30—60 minutes*).

   Walking Meditation (in nature if possible) / Assimilation period (as long as you need).

5. **Clear out your retreat space, leave no trace.**

6. **Close retreat with a bow, expressing gratitude for the teachers and students who came before us.**

ONE FINAL NOTE BEFORE BEGINNING A RETREAT

WE CANNOT PRACTICE MEDITATION, relax all day, and wish our daily lives were always like that. We always come back to the real world. We must accept that we need to work and engage in our communities. Even the hermits of old came back to civilization. Treating our retreat experience as separate from our regular lives *is* spiritual materialism. Retreating is not a template for a new life; it is a practice. Take full advantage of the time you set aside for your retreat, and let whatever is waiting for you sit patiently until your return. Stay present.

When we first add retreating to our spiritual path, it's normal to feel that the transition back to the real world is a bit abrasive. It can be drastic, especially if we have successfully de-stressed and are feeling refreshed, to feel an emotional switch flipped as we return to our responsibilities. But that is precisely why we must retreat! We must get enough space to experience that difference, that gap between our potential for meditation and our actual experience. That is where we need to do the work.

We are not in control of all of our circumstances, but we have the power to maintain our meditation in all of our actions. Retreating gets us back to basics, giving us an opportunity to review precisely how we are living. It shows us where our energy gravitates when we have no agenda. It helps us dial in on what is important, what helps us thrive, and shines a light on who we love. With the clarity gained from retreating, we can begin to review where we use our energy wisely and where we may be better off adjusting our method. We may not be able to plan weekly retreats, but we can recognize when we are in meditation and when our emotional triggers take us out of meditation.

As we learn better strategies to maintain ourselves, we reduce the need to retreat from the world as often. Retreating can always serve as a space for reflection–even annual ones set around birthdays are a great way to reflect on the specifics of life and what has changed since your last contemplation. No matter how financially successful we may be or how much we may be living our dreams, each of us needs to routinely come back to the beginning, shed what is not working for us, and rebirth ourselves in the same skin but with refreshed perspective. Retreating can be the reset button, but we must create good, regular habits that maintain our meditation. Regardless of where you are starting from, I hope that this work can help you find the space necessary to walk through life more peacefully and meaningfully.

Take a deep inhale through your nose and into your belly. Pause for a moment, then exhale out your mouth with a soft *ahhhhhh*. A deep breath is always available to us before we proceed with our actions. May this guide to the retreat experience serve you well.

GOOD LUCK!

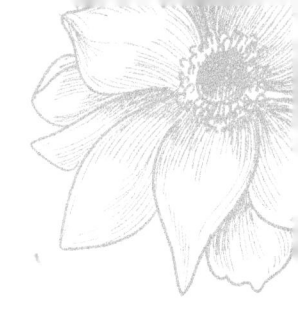

APPENDIX II

RECOMMENDED RESOURCES

I INTENTIONALLY DID MY best not to bog down the text with statistics and proofs of theory. But that does not mean that this book was not heavily researched. Although I have benefited personally from all the advice shared, I can claim little of it as my own. It is the advice of the great teachers in my life, including neuroscientists, spiritual leaders, and my parents and schoolteachers, in my own words. My hope was that this book would serve as a template for your journey and a catalyst to laser in on what needs your attention. The following resources were the source materials for better understanding our brains, where many of the themes for well-being and spiritual practice overlap.

It can be difficult to sort things into neat categories when everything is so integrated—but I have done my best. I have presented these materials in order of their references within this book. It is more important to find voices that inspire you than to read everything out there, and the following teachers are the ones who spoke clearest to me and, hopefully, to you as well.

HONESTY

Cutting Through Spiritual Materialism, Chögyam Trungpa Rinpoche

You Are Here, Thich Nhat Hahn

The End of Your World, Adyashanti

Meditation in Action, Chögyam Trungpa Rinpoche

Things You Can See Only When You Slow Down, Haemin Sunim

Buddha's Brain, Rick Hanson

Buddhism Without Beliefs, Stephen Batchelor

The Science of Enlightenment, Shinzen Young (the book is good, but the lecture series is so much better!)

Neuro Dharma, Rick Hanson

NOURISHMENT

Gut, Guilia Enders

The Plant Paradox, Dr. Stephen Gundry

Food Rules, Michael Pollan

The Third Plate, Dan Barber

The End of Overeating, David A. Kessler, MD

Eating Animals, Jonathan Safran Foer

Food Politics, Marion Nestle

RECOMMENDED RESOURCES

How to Cook Your Life, Kosho Uchiyama

Hardcore Zen, Brad Warner

Salt Fat Acid Heat, Samin Nosrat

REST

The Science of Sleep, John Medina (lecture)

Grow a New Body, Dr. Alberto Villoldo

Your Best Brain, John Medina (lecture series)

Hardwiring Happiness, Rick Hanson

Brain Rules, John Medina

Dream Yoga, Andrew Holechek

EXERCISE

The Longevity Plan: Seven Lessons from Ancient China, Dr. John Day, Jane Ann Day, and Matthew LaPlante

The Comfort Crisis, Michael Easter

Moving Toward Balance: 8 Weeks of Yoga with Rodney Yee, Rodney Yee and Nina Zolotov

Inner Engineering, Sadguru

Perfectly Imperfect, John Baptiste

The Four Desires, Rod Stryker

Light on Life, BKS Iyengar

One Simple Thing, Eddie Stern

MEDITATION

The Secrets of Meditation, davidji

The Mind Illuminated, Culadasa (John Yates)

The Path to Insight Meditation, Joseph Goldstein

The Path Is the Goal, Chögyam Trungpa Rinpoche

The Gradual Path, Miles Neale (audiobook)

10% Happier, Dan Harris

Progressive Stages of Meditation on Emptiness, Khenpo Tsultrim Gyamtso Rinpoche

Getting Unstuck, Pema Chödrön

CURIOSITY

Habits of a Happy Brain, Loretta Graziano Breuning

The Science of Positivity, Loretta Graziano Breuning

The River of Consciousness, Dr. Oliver Sacks

This Is Your Brain on Music, Daniel J. Levitin

The Art of Making Memories, Meik Wiking

The Lost Art of Reading Nature Signs, Tristan Gooley

Forest Bathing, Dr. Qing Li

RELATIONSHIPS

The Craving Mind, Judson Brewer

The Empath's Survival Guide, Dr. Judith Orloff

How Emotions Are Made, Lisa Feldman Barrett

Boundaries and Protection, Pixie Lighthorse

Radical Self-Acceptance, Tara Brach

The Life-Changing Magic of Tidying Up, Marie Kondo

The Art of Happiness, His Holiness the Dalai Lama

Anger, Thich Nhat Hahn

The Wisdom of the Shamans, Don Jose Ruiz

The Art of Solitude, Stephen Batchelor

RESPONSIBILITY

Work, Sex, Money, Chögyam Trungpa Rinpoche

The Four Agreements, Don Miguel Ruiz

Training the Mind, Chögyam Trungpa Rinpoche

Man's Search for Meaning, Viktor Frankl

Awakening from the Daydream, David Nichtern

Don't Be a Jerk, Brad Warner

The Tao of Leadership, John Heider

The Art of Simple Living, Shunmyo Masuno

ACCEPTANCE

The Untethered Soul, Michael A. Singer

The Wisdom of Insecurity, Alan Watts

Fail, Fail Again, Fail Better, Pema Chödrön

Be Here Now, Ram Dass

The Surrender Experiment, Michael A. Singer

What Is This?, Martine and Stephen Batchelor

The Subtle Art of Not Giving a F**k, Mark Manson

GENEROSITY

After the Ecstasy, the Laundry, Jack Kornfield

Living Beautifully, Pema Chödrön

Real Love, Sharon Salzberg

Smile at Fear, Chögyam Trungpa Rinpoche

A Heart Full of Peace, Joseph Goldstein

Love for Imperfect Things, Haemin Sunim

Why Buddhism Is True, Robert Wright

After Buddhism, Stephen Batchelor

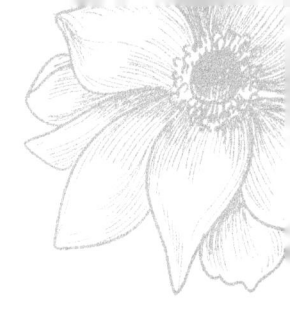

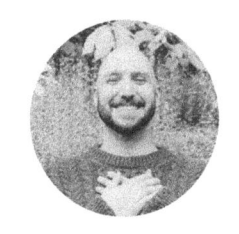

ABOUT THE AUTHOR

JOHNNY SCIFO IS AN E-RYT-500 advanced certified yoga and meditation teacher and has been a devoted yogi for nearly two decades. Trained in diverse healing modalities, his energy practices and multi-instrumental sound healing invoke powerful experiences for his students. A mixture of modern science, ancient wisdom, and raw love, Johnny is a living example of the internal power we each possess for positive change and the ability to fulfill one's dreams and dharma. He has led thousands of students through yoga festivals, retreats, and sharing his take on meditation, music, and neuroscience with educators in both academia and spiritual circles, including Lululemon, Kripalu, the Rubin Museum, Ramapo College, and SUNY New Paltz. He is an active contributor to Insight Timer, inspiring over one million meditations worldwide with his healing music and holistic approach to modern living.

MORE FROM JOHNNY

Awakening course, free meditations, and playlists at: **www.johnnyscifo.com**

LEAVE A REVIEW!

For a self-published author like myself, reviews mean the world! So, please, leave a review on the platform from which you purchased the book. I read every one!